Nursing Curriculum

Development, Structure, Function

Freda S. Scales, R.N., Ph.D.

Dean, College of Nursing
Valparaiso University
Valparaiso, Indiana

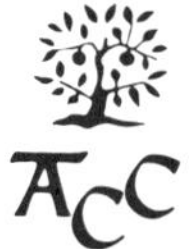

APPLETON-CENTURY-CROFTS/Norwalk, Connecticut

ISBN - 0-8385-7021-6

Notice: The author(s) and publisher of this volume have taken care that the information and recommendations contained herein are accurate and compatible with the standards generally accepted at the time of publication.

85 86 87 88 / 10 9 8 7 6 5 4 3 2 1

Prentice-Hall International, Inc., London
Prentice-Hall of Australia, Pty. Ltd., Sydney
Prentice-Hall Canada, Inc.
Prentice-Hall of India Private Limited, New Delhi
Prentice-Hall of Japan, Inc., Tokyo
Prentice-Hall of Southeast Asia (Pte.) Ltd., Singapore
Whitehall Books Ltd., Wellington, New Zealand
Editora Prentice-Hall do Brasil Ltda., Rio de Janeiro

Library of Congress Cataloging in Publication Data

Scales, Freda S.
Nursing curriculum.

Includes index.
1. Nursing—Study and teaching. 2. Nursing schools—Curricula. 3. Curriculum planning.
I. Title. [DNLM: 1. Curriculum. 2. Education, Nursing. WY 18 S281n]
RT73.S28 1984 610.73'07'11 84-12462
ISBN 0-8385-7021-6

Design: Lynn M. Luchetti

PRINTED IN THE UNITED STATES OF AMERICA

Contents

Preface

Curriculum development is constant, just like growth and development. It can occur haphazardly or systematically; be planned or unplanned. *Nursing Curriculum: Development, Structure, Function* demonstrates how curriculum development can be systematic and planned. It provides the faculty member involved in curriculum planning or the graduate student in a nursing curriculum course with a method and rationale for the development and structure and an understanding of the function of a nursing curriculum.

The tool for curriculum planning in this text is an evaluation model, specifically the CIPP model of Stufflebeam. Any comprehensive program evaluation model would be appropriate, for the purpose of the models is for judgments to be made about the contextual framework of a program, the resources available, the weaknesses and strengths of its implementation and operation, and its effectiveness to the consumer. When these concerns are addressed, a curriculum has been developed, implemented, and evaluated.

It is hoped that the reader develops a sense of order for curricular planning but also a sense of flexibility. Virtually nothing in this world is 100 percent orderly or perfect. People are the planners and operators of a curriculum, which guarantees a lack of extreme order and predictability of results. Following a plan in curriculum planning, however, does enable idiosyncratic people to produce a fairly consensual, operational curriculum.

Writing this text has been difficult. I taught a course in nursing curriculum for 7 years and when I began writing, I thought that all I would have to do would be to put my lecture notes in writing. Two years after starting this project, my "lecture notes" have been manipulated so much that I would be hard pressed to find them in the text. When I lecture, I can talk in phrases and choppy sentences; I can drag out articles for direct reference to illustrate a point. When writing a book, the sentences must become grammatically correct and the literature review has to become readable instead of accessible. This task was almost more than I could do or even wanted to bear. There were those who did make the task bearable, however; Dick Baepler eloquated my English and Marie Cahn lifted up my prepositions out of the miry clay. A special acknowledgment is given to Arline Phipps for becoming permanently glued to the word processor.

Final acknowledgments could also be in the form of a dedication: to my faculty peers at Indiana University who influenced my curricular thoughts through discussion, and sometimes heated arguments for 13 years; to graduate students in the nursing curriculum classes for looking puzzled after I thought I had said something quite profound; and to a faculty for whom I am now Dean, who is very strong and independent. "Thank you" seems trite, but thank you it is, for without all of the events mentioned in this acknowledgment section, I would still be staring at disorganized lecture notes.

Nursing Curriculum

Development, Structure, Function

1

Introduction

One way of developing a curriculum is with the guidance of an evaluation model, such as seen in Steele (1978) and Clark et al. (1983). That is the approach taken in this text; Stufflebeam's model of program evaluation (CIPP) is used as a guide to plan a curriculum (context evaluation), structure a curriculum (input evaluation), implement a curriculum (process evaluation), and recycle or evaluate a curriculum (product evaluation) (Worthen and Sanders, 1973).

At the conclusion of each unit, an example of the particular evaluation component (*c*ontext, *i*nput, *p*rocess, *p*roduct—CIPP) just completed is presented and questions are asked that when answered will provide data for the evaluation; sources are given as to where data can be acquired.

MODEL FOR CURRICULAR DEVELOPMENT

Planning and Structuring Decisions

Planning decisions involve the establishment of the philosophy, objectives, and framework of the program. Within the philosophic, behavioral, and conceptual framework, the design and structure of the curriculum take shape. Decisions for curricular structuring include determining what the resources are or should be for the implementation of the curriculum. Data are collected regarding faculty and facility availability, student characteristics, and proposed faculty–student ratios.

Implementing Decisions

Implementation decisions determine how the curriculum will actually be carried out within the curriculum design. They involve judgments concerning such matters as credit allocation, sequencing of courses, course titles, faculty allocation, and student enrollment.

Recycling Decisions

Recycling decisions are based on the continuous curricular evaluation process and may result in a determination of the need for change. The assessed need for change returns faculty full circle to planning evaluation in order to determine the type of change needed and thereby the planning required for a revised curriculum. Because of the systematic method of evaluation, curricular development is systematic and continuous and decisions regarding the need for change will be systematic and continuous.

GOVERNANCE AND FACULTY ORGANIZATION

The shaping of the curriculum is very much the special province of the faculty. The faculty's sense of ownership of the curriculum clearly influences its effectiveness in attaining the goals of the educational program. The last chapter discusses various faculty governance designs and approaches, all of which influence the development, implementation, and evaluation of the curriculum.

CURRICULUM: DEVELOPMENT, STRUCTURE, FUNCTION

Each time a curricular component is devised, it is examined from the standpoint of its development, structure, and function. Faculty's development of each curricular component is influenced by the student/learner, the setting, the society, and the subject matter (Bevis, 1982; Chater, 1975; Tyler, 1950). Since these influences converge in interrelated ways in curricular considerations, they are viewed, whenever possible, from the perspective of their integrative character.

The structure is what the curricular component actually looks like. Is it a diagram? A paragraph? What does it have "in it" after it has been developed? What does a conceptual framework or a curricular organizer look like?

The function is the curricular purpose of the component. Now that the faculty has developed a philosophy, what does it do in the curriculum itself? What does it do to and for the faculty?

Development Sequences

Ideally, faculty involved in curricular development or revision should start at the logical beginning of the process as is suggested in the sequences of chapters in this text. In actual fact, however, curricular development and revisions may begin at any point in the sequence and with any element of the curriculum. Actually, it is probably very wise to develop and revise a curriculum first and then write or rewrite the philosophy, for by the time the curriculum has been revised by faculty, its philosophy has been clarified through discussion of concrete and specific issues and therefore is far simpler to agree upon and express. The same can be said about outcomes or objectives. Oftentimes faculty finds that it has over time revised the curriculum to the point that the objectives need updating to be congruent with the previous revisions.

In a text such as this, or in a curriculum course, the content is necessarily sequenced for learning purposes, but in actual practice, development and implementation of the curriculum is an integrated phenomenon and therefore is developed in a very integrated, interrelating manner; one component will not necessarily spring "full grown" and naturally from another, nor will any single component usually stand without some revision after subsequent parts are developed. The philosophy may be influenced as objectives are developed, and objectives may change as the conceptual framework expands and contracts. In effect then, curricular development has no beginning or end, no real starting or stopping point, and certainly no "perfect product," even when the final faculty meeting is adjourned.

What the author hopes the reader develops as a result of reading this text is a perspective on curriculum development that values curricular coherence together with a broad flexibility in achieving that coherence. In curricular development, the fact that faculty and students are creative individuals must be taken into account. A curriculum will not be acceptable if it lacks recognition of human flexibilities, idiosyncracies, individualism, and creativity.

REFERENCES

Bevis, E. *Curriculum Building in Nursing—A Process* (3rd ed.). St. Louis: C.V. Mosby, 1982.

Chater, S. A conceptual framework for curriculum development. *Nurs Outlook*, 1975, 23, 428–433.

Clark, T., Goodwin, M., Mariani, M., et al: Curriculum evaluation: An application of Stufflebeam's model in a baccalaureate school of nursing. *J Nurs Educ*, 1983, 22, 54–58.

Steele, S. *Educational Evaluation in Nursing*. U.S.A.: Slack, 1978.

Tyler, R. W. *Basic Principles of Curriculum and Instruction*. Chicago: The University of Chicago, 1950.

Worthen, B. R., & Sanders, J. R. *Educational Evaluation: Theory and Practice*. Worthington, Ohio: Charles A. Jones, 1973.

Unit 1

CONTEXT EVALUATION FOR PLANNING DECISIONS

The philosophy, conceptual framework, and curricular objectives form the framework for the curriculum. Context evaluation consists of collecting information on beliefs about nursing, education, and existence; concepts prominent in forming the discipline and subject matter of nursing; and behaviors appropriate to and required of the graduate.

Curricular planning decisions are vacuous without a belief system, subject matter, and behaviors to be developed.

2

Philosophy

The philosophic basis of a curriculum is the creation and property of faculty, even though it is abstractly seen as "the school's philosophy." There are many influences on the faculty as it develops a philosophic base that in turn permeates and influences the curriculum.

DEVELOPMENT

Faculty

Without a doubt, faculty members come to a program already holding to a general philosophy or set of beliefs about the world in general and more specifically about education and nursing. Packer (1979) identified three major philosophic attitudes found among most faculty members: realism, pragmatism, and idealism. Realism emphasizes what exists and what is real in an immediate, verifiable sense. Faculty members with a realistic philosophy "are concerned with facts and an established body of knowledge for the basis for their program's curriculum" (Packer, 1979, p. 48). The body of knowledge is based on empiric data and research. Pragmatic faculty members "believe that knowledge is always changing and that the student should have the opportunity to learn that which attracts him and has meaning for him" (Packer, 1979, p. 48). The curriculum of the pragmatists is heavily influenced by the consumer and the trends of the profession. Faculty members who profess an idealistic philosophy "place emphasis on ideas. They believe that the students need to find order in the information that is available" (Packer, 1979, p. 48). The curriculum of the idealists is a search for truth in ideas, which may not necessarily be "real" or "pragmatic."

Surveying or pooling the faculty's beliefs is a useful step in the development of the philosophy of a program. A study by Miller (1979) showed that the majority of one surveyed school's nursing faculty held a pragmatic philosophy of life and education more than a realistic, idealistic or existential philosophy. The surveying and pooling get to the general philosophic bent of the faculty and may help faculty by giving it a springboard from which to begin to develop a broad, consensual philosophic position.

Institutional

Constraining, molding, and further guiding the faculty's philosophy that serves as the belief basis of the nursing program is the influence of the philosophic constraints of the nursing program's sponsoring institution. If the institution is denominational, then the philosophic foundation for the curriculum and its development will be influenced by that denomination's philosophy and belief. Likewise, if the institution is state-owned or assisted, then the philosophic position will necessarily be broad, global, and perhaps even vague in order to reflect the pluralism of the people of the state who are supporting the program through state revenue.

Method

With each faculty member's own philosophy and the institution's philosophy as major constraints or influences, the faculty develops, writes, and establishes a philosophy or set of belief statements that underlies and serves as a basis for the program's curriculum. The development and writing of a philosophy are usually done either by a small ad hoc committee or by one person, after having received input from the whole faculty. Whatever the method, the document is approved by all faculty members, indicating their agreement that it indeed is the working philosophic foundation of the curriculum, and thereby able to influence something as grand as a curriculum conceptual base and something as small (but not insignificant) as a day's clinical focus.

As mentioned in the introduction, just because it is sequentially first in curriculum exhibits and is indeed the philosophic basis for the program, the final philosophic statement need not be completed and established first in the process of curricular development and revision. Some philosophic jottings and brain storming with faculty must necessarily occur when initiating a program or contemplating revisions of an existing program, but completing and establishing the philosophy may occur after much of the curriculum is developed. The latter approach may be more appropriate for the faculty since the process of curricular development will itself draw out key philosophic issues requiring the faculty to face them and thus to develop a more common mind. When a program is already in existence, curricular components may be revised, retroactively necessitating a change in the written philosophy; typically, the curricular change starts from an informal but consensual philosophic change or new awareness within the faculty, with the change instigating a revision in the philosophic document, not vice versa.

Human beings are goal directed.

Nursing is goal directed.

Health is an optimal state of being.

TRUTH statement with ACTION statements:

Human beings, being goal directed, strive for an optimal state of well-being. The nursing profession exists to assist the individual to attain the highest potential for her/his state of being.

Figure 1. Truth statements.

STRUCTURE

What does a philosophic statement look like? According to Rokeach (1968), a philosophy contains a belief statement followed by an action statement. The belief can be expressed as something true or false (truth), good or bad (evaluative), and/or as something that should or should not exist (exhortative) (Figs. 1, 2, and 3).

Nursing education programs usually have all three kinds of belief statements at some point or another in their philosophies. Faculty do not

The nursing profession benefits society.

It is of benefit to society to strive for an optimal state of well-being.

It is good when health is viewed as an optimal state of well-being.

EVALUATIVE statement with ACTION statements:

It is of benefit to human beings when nursing assists them to their optimal state of well-being.

Figure 2. Evaluative statements.

Nursing should assist society in its striving for health restoration, maintenance or promotion.

It is imperative that human beings are recognized as unique and idiosyncratic.

Health must be recognized as being on a continuum.

EXHORTATIVE statements with ACTION statements:

Because health should be viewed as on a continuum and individuals as unique and idiosyncratic, nurses should assist society along the health care continuum of health restoration, maintenance and/or promotion.

Figure 3. Exhortative statements.

always add an action statement, however, so frequently the "philosophy" of a nursing program is actually a compilation of faculty's belief statements of truths, exhortations, and evaluations, to use Rokeach's categories (Fig. 4).

Whatever the shape and character of the final philosophic document, through it the faculty expresses its collective views on the main features

Exhortative: Health should be a right, not a privilege.

Truth: Human beings are unique and idiosyncratic.

Evaluative: It is good for the society that the nursing profession exists.

TRUTH, EXHORTATIVE, AND EVALUATIVE statements with ACTION statements:

Since nursing recognizes that health is a right, not a privilege, each individual in the health care system, regardless of his/her idiosyncracies, will benefit because of the nursing profession's position as client advocate.

Figure 4. Truth, Exhortative, and Evaluative statements.

of the educational process. These include the concepts that usually constitute the subject matter of nursing (humankind, health, nursing, and possibly environment), the learner in the program, and perhaps the type of program, such as associate (technical) or baccalaureate (professional).

Subject Matter

HUMANKIND

Humankind is often designated in the philosophy as Man, Society, or Individual–Family–Community. Faculty's beliefs usually result in statements about a unitary, holistic, developmental, adaptative, or compartmentalized (biologic, sociologic, psychological, and spiritual) person who exists within a realistic, pragmatic, or idealistic framework.

The following are examples of belief statements made in a philosophic framework. A different belief statement was used with a different philosophic framework for each example to demonstrate many of the possible permutations. A philosophy may indeed be all one type of belief statement, e.g., truths, in one philosophic framework, e.g., pragmatism, but the likelihood of that is slim (Table 1).

HEALTH

Faculty's beliefs about health may be quite varied and cause more conflict than any of the other elements of the philosophy. The beliefs may be that health is holistic, a feeling of well-being, a statement of optimum physical function, that health is on a continuum between illness and wellness, or a combination of the above, such as contained in the World Health Organization's definition of health. Whatever the belief statement, it is the consensus of the faculty's concept of health, and as such, serves as the foundation for what is included in the program in relation to health (Table 2).

TABLE 1. BELIEF STATEMENTS ABOUT HUMAN BEINGS

Belief Statement	Philosophic Framework	Statements
Truth	Realistic	Individuals are bio-psycho-social beings.
Exhortative	Pragmatic	Individuals should be viewed as idiosyncratic beings with common needs.
Evaluative	Idealistic	Human beings value the search for truth.
Truth	Realistic with Action Statement	Humankind is composed of bio-psycho-social beings and therefore is able to yield empiric data.

TABLE 2. BELIEF STATEMENTS ABOUT HEALTH

Belief Statement	Philosophic Framework	Statements
Truth	Pragmatic	Health is the present state of being.
Exhortative	Idealistic	Health should be a right, not a privilege.
Evaluative	Realistic	Health is valued by human beings.
Evaluative	Realistic with Action Statement	Because human beings value health, they will comply with health restoration, maintenance, and promotion regimens.

NURSING

What does the faculty believe about nursing? Bevis (1982) suggests that there have been four major philosophic bases of nursing to which faculty adhered at some point in history: asceticism (self-denial and duty), romanticism (service), pragmatism (functional), and humanistic existentialism (holism). Whether it adopts one of the above beliefs or a combination thereof, the faculty develops a belief statement related to nursing which becomes the philosophic basis of the nursing content in the educational program (Table 3).

ENVIRONMENT

Oftentimes the faculty's belief about the environment is embedded in its statement about society or humankind because of a belief in an interactive relationship between persons and the environment. There are some faculty members, however, who value the environmental concept sufficiently to believe that it warrants a separate philosophic statement and therefore include one in the philosophy of their program. One frequently found expression about environment stresses its reciprocal influence on

TABLE 3. BELIEF STATEMENTS ABOUT NURSING

Belief Statement	Philosophic Framework	Statements
Truth	Realistic	Nursing is a service-oriented discipline (asceticism) (Bevis, 1982).
Exhortative	Pragmatic	Nursing has a definite role in the health care of society (pragmaticism) (Bevis, 1982).
Evaluative	Idealistic	Nursing is valued by society because of its unique humanistic therapeutic interventions (humanistic existentialism) (Bevis, 1982).
Truth	Realistic with Action Statement	Nursing is a service-oriented discipline and it only exists as long as society needs it.

TABLE 4. BELIEF STATEMENTS ABOUT ENVIRONMENT

Belief Statement	Philosophic Framework	Statements
Truth	Realistic	The environment controls people's behavior.
Exhortative	Pragmatic	Depending upon the circumstances, it must be recognized that it is always the external or internal environment of human beings that influences behavior.
Evaluative	Idealistic	The environment and the individual have a reciprocal relationship.
Evaluative	Idealistic with Action Statement	The environment and the individual have a reciprocal relationship, thereby creating a holistic framework of existence.

and relationship with human beings. An additional view that is often found in these statements distinguishes between an internal and an external environment in man and society (Table 4).

Learner

Faculty often expresses its views about the learner and learning, since it is developing belief statements related to an educational program. Sometimes these views are subsumed under the statement regarding humankind but often they are expressed at a separate place. Frequently faculty beliefs concerning the learner or learning are eclectic: they believe learning is associational at times, cognitive at times, and affective or subjective at other times, while often taking place in various combinations simultaneously.

Faculty's belief about learning is influenced by its basic general philosophy. For the pragmatist, learning should be the acquisition of what is existent for immediate preparation for practice; the realist believes that learning should be the acquisition of as much material, facts, and concepts as possible; for the idealist, learning is a search for truth of the essence (uniqueness) of nursing and may lean more toward the theoretic (Table 5).

Education Program

Faculty may want to express its belief about nursing education. The faculty's belief determines the value placed on the type of program and therefore how it is to be conducted. For example, if faculty believes that nurses have multiple roles and require a professional education but it teaches in a program whose purpose is that of graduating within 2 years nurses whose primary role is that of a "care-giver" (Kramer, 1981), conflict may occur in the implementation of the curriculum. A clear understand-

TABLE 5. BELIEF STATEMENTS ABOUT LEARNING

Belief Statement	Philosophic Framework	Statements
Truth	Pragmatic	Learning in a nursing education program is for the acquisition and development of skills and abilities with a high utilization value.
Exhortative	Idealistic	Learning must be a continuous process in a profession that is constantly researching for a better way of health care.
Evaluative	Realistic	Learning is only valuable if it contains not only the cognitive and psychomotor domains but the affective as well.
Exhortative	Idealistic with Action Statement	Learning must be a continuous process in the nursing profession so that the consumer will always benefit from the latest in a series of consistently improving developments.

ing among faculty members as to what type of program (technical or professional) is in place and a philosophic statement regarding the same may help to alleviate later conflicts (Table 6).

FUNCTION

The major function of the philosophy is to provide a belief system or philosophic foundation that supports the purpose of the program and provides a framework for the curriculum. Packer (1979) has taken three philosophies and threaded them through curriculum components to il-

TABLE 6. BELIEF STATEMENTS ABOUT NURSING EDUCATION

Belief Statement	Philosophic Framework	Statements
Truth	Idealistic	Nursing education is the avenue in which the discipline is developed.
Exhortative	Realistic	Nursing education must provide as complete a complement of learning activities as is possible in a given time.
Evaluative	Pragmatic	The value of nursing education is seen in the marketing of the graduate.
Exhortative	Realistic	Nursing education must provide as complete a complement of learning activities as is possible in a given time so that when placed into practice the graduate is as fully prepared as can be expected.

Components	i	ii	iii
Philosophy	Realist	Idealist	Pragmatist
Curriculum	Special subjects	Integrated	Undifferentiated
Objectives	Behavioral and instructional	Goals and objectives	Goals and contracts
Learning	Behaviorist	Nonbehaviorist—some cognitivists	Cognitivists (Third forcers)
Teaching	Teacher-centered lectures	Teacher–Student lecture and discussion	Student-centered inquiry/discovery
Evaluation	Objective	Objectives and written (essays and papers)	Projects and papers

Figure 5. Curriculum consistency; curriculum options. *(Reprinted from the Journal of Nursing Education, April 1979, Vol. 18, No. 4, p. 48. Published by SLACK Incorporated, Medical Publishers, copyright 1979.)*

lustrate how different philosophies influence the curriculum in nursing programs (Fig. 5).

Table 7 shows an example of belief and philosophic statements framed within one statement-type (truth) and one philosophy (realism).

The function of the consensual or, perhaps in most cases, compromised philosophy of the faculty is to provide a belief system on which to base the curriculum and all other aspects of the nursing program.

PROGRAM AIMS

A statement of the program's purpose or aims may be placed adjacent to the philosophy, particularly following the belief statement about the program. The formulation is usually succinct and concise, informing the reader, based on the philosophy of the faculty, of the purpose of the program. An example of the purpose of a professional program at a baccalaureate level might be to provide the community (nation) with professional nurses for health care delivery. Additional aims of the program might be to provide an environment for nursing research in the community as well as opportunities for continuing education for professionals within the community.

TABLE 7. STATEMENTS WITHIN ONE BELIEF TYPE AND ONE PHILOSOPHIC FRAMEWORK

Belief Statement	Philosophic Framework	Statements
Truth	Realistic	Individuals are bio-psycho-social beings.
Truth	Realistic	Health is on a continuum of illness to wellness.
Truth	Realistic	Nursing is a process in a goal-directed framework.
Truth	Realistic	The environment is a controlling factor on people's behavior.
Truth	Realistic	Learning involves the cognitive, psychomotor, and affective domains, sometimes separately, but most of the time simultaneously.
Truth	Realistic	Nursing education in the baccalaureate program is the provision of a full complement of learning activities for the preparation of the professional nurse.
Truth	Realistic with Action Statement	Since individuals are bio-psycho-social beings, they are at all times at some point of health, since health is at any point on an illness to wellness continuum. With the environment being an influencing factor in human beings' behavior, nursing (part of the environment) influences individuals by way of the nursing process to attain goals of health within that continuum—restoration, maintenance or promotion.
		Since people are bio-psycho-social beings, the cognitive (thinking), affective (emotions), and psychomotor (motor) domains are affected in each learning activity and experience of the learner. Baccalaureate nursing education is the provision of the fullest complement of affective, psychomotor, and cognitive learning activities as is possible for the preparation of the professional nurse.

REFERENCES

Bevis, E. *Curriculum Building in Nursing—A Process* (3rd ed.). St. Louis: C. V. Mosby, 1982.

Kramer, M. Philosophical foundations of baccalaureate nursing education. *Nurs Outlook*, 1981, 29, 224–338.

Miller, C. *Measurement of faculty's philosophical orientation at Indiana University School of Nursing*. Unpublished manuscript, 1979.

Packer, J. Curriculum consistency. *J Nurs Educ*, 1979, 18, 47–52.

Rokeach, M. *Beliefs, Attitudes, Values*. San Francisco: Jossey-Bass, 1968.

3

Curricular Framework

The framework of a curriculum reflects the program's philosophy in that it further develops key philosophic concepts such as humankind, health, and nursing by defining and relating them. The interrelationship of the concepts is the basic, skeletal organizational framework of the curriculum. As the concepts are further defined within the framework, the curriculum becomes established. Course titles, lesson plans, clinical activities, and behavioral objectives all reflect the organizational framework. The function of the conceptual framework is to provide a rationale for the selection of learning activities and a structure for ordering and sequencing content to produce a unified whole (Wu, 1979).

REASONS FOR A CONCEPTUAL CURRICULAR FRAMEWORK

A conceptual framework promotes a conceptual approach to learning. The learner is unable to assimilate vast amounts of knowledge but can internalize and understand concepts which subsume many facts too cumbersome to memorize. Learning concepts is "meaningful learning" (Ausubel, 1968; Bartlett, 1932); learning facts is memorized, rote learning. Since the occurrence of the "knowledge explosion," the student can no longer learn all the accumulating facts. An analysis of the content provides those fundamental ideas or concepts that form the structure (framework) of the discipline (nursing) to be learned and taught (Posner, 1976). By learning within this structure, the student acquires the essence of the discipline in the most economic manner, without having to learn every one of the facts subsumed by each basic concept.

Two types of concepts are primarily used in the structures or frameworks representing nursing: class concepts and propositional statements. A class concept is one that selects a group or set of things or events (facts) as instances of the same kind of thing (concept) because they share common properties (Posner, 1976). Humankind is an example of a class

Class Concept:	**Human Kind**
Set of things:	Females Males
Sharing common properties:	Biologic
	Psychological
	Spiritual
	Sociologic
	Physical

Figure 6. Class concept: Humankind.

concept. Humankind as a class concept represents women and men of all shapes, sizes, personalities, and ages. Biologic, psychological, spiritual, sociologic, and physical attributes of women and men are the common properties that place them within the class of humankind (Fig. 6).

A proposition is a combination or relationship of concepts that asserts something (conceptual framework) (Posner, 1976). The framework permits teaching the basic concepts prior to the proposition that the concepts support (inductive) or teaching the proposition prior to the concepts that the proposition explains (deductive) or a combination thereof. An example of a proposition statement that serves as a "relational concept" (Huckabay, 1980, p. 103) is a conceptual framework. A conceptual framework takes concepts (health, society, nursing) and relates them to each other.

Propositional Statement (Conceptual Framework):
In nursing, professionals interact with human beings in order to promote restoration, maintenance and/or health.

Planned sequences of content and learning activities in the curriculum enable the student to focus on the relationships between the concepts of the proposition in a simple to complex development. The framework provides structure and organization on which to build and develop a logical curriculum in nursing education. The framework or curriculum organizer is conceptual rather than theoretic because there are no settled theories of nursing from which to build a curriculum or a practice. Concepts of human beings, nursing, and health, generally accepted and loosely interrelated by faculty, serve as a framework for a curriculum and enable the development, structuring, and teaching of nursing content.

WHY HAVE A CONCEPTUAL FRAMEWORK?

But why does the faculty need to develop a curriculum that has a logical order? Why do content and learning activities need to be based on an interrelated whole? Why cannot faculty teach courses that are "germane" to nursing—nursing practice, the nursing profession—without fitting them into some kind of structure? Good questions and well-worn ones. The consumer of the curriculum (human beings/society) is whole. The practice of the graduate is whole, purposeful. Up until recently educators have allowed, even required the graduate to form her own wholeness—gestalt, of the society, persons, nursing, and health relationship. The nature of this end product is largely unknown since little, if any, research has shown what framework a practitioner actually has in his or her practice. With the advent of nursing theory and model development has come the realization that indeed nursing could be structured in a meaningful reality. It has become clear that the discipline of nursing is not just the fortuitous end result of a compilation of courses. Content and learning activities began to be developed within the framework of society/persons, nursing, and health relationships, rather than in a disease and medical orientation. With the realization that human beings, the consumer, and nursing are (w)holistic, it was natural that the curriculum of this profession become (w)holistic. Hence we now see in nursing education the advent of the "integrated" curriculum—the attempt to present to the student a perspective on the whole—the whole of its consumer (persons in society) and the whole of itself (human beings–health–nursing). "Integration" in most cases, however, has been a bastardized organization of content and learning activities which had been traditionally taught in nursing programs. Organizing, framing, and integrating a curriculum is not synonymous with the disintegration of valid nursing content and learning activities; it is, rather, synonymous with sequencing and building content on and within a framework in order to graduate a practitioner cognizant of the interrelatedness of her or his profession with human beings and health.

DEVELOPING A CONCEPTUAL FRAMEWORK

The conceptual framework should be consistent with the belief statements of society, nursing, and health in the philosophy. The framework provides definitions of the concepts, definitions that are further developed in the courses comprising the curriculum.

DEVELOPMENT

The development of the curriculum's framework or organizational structure occurs after faculty decides its beliefs or philosophy about the major concepts (human beings, health, nursing) that will be the basis of the curriculum (Hall, 1979). The conceptual framework will have definitions of the concepts and attributes or subconcepts. Faculty will find it can define the major concepts in a number of ways, either within the framework of the many nursing models or by way of an eclectic interpretation of its own. All definitions, regardless of the framework or model, reflect the basic beliefs expressed in the program's philosophy.

Survey results of baccalaureate and masters' programs responding to questions about their conceptual frameworks indicated that baccalaureate programs were using the established theorists (Orem, Rogers, Levine, Kind, Roy, and Johnson) to some degree in describing the major concepts (Hall, 1979). Forty-one percent of the baccalaureate programs surveyed based their concept definitions on one or more of the theorists. "Only in rare instances in any of the programs however, where a particular theorist's framework was largely used, was the framework employed without modification particular to the individual program" (Hall, 1979, p. 28).

Hall (1979) asked faculty in nursing programs to identify the activities included in making its decision about a framework. The most frequently used activities were "(1) review of the literature, followed by (2) informal discussion with the faculty at the school, and (3) establishment of committees" (Hall, 1979, p. 28). Activities which were seldom identified as being part of the decision-making process included such things as "systematic collection of data from other schools, discussions with representatives from area schools, and reviewing the frameworks in area schools" (Hall, 1979, p. 28).

Concept Identification

Nursing, health, human beings, and environment appear to be the most prominent concepts identified by faculty to represent and frame the nursing curriculum in nursing programs. Newman traced the four concepts of health, client, nursing, and environment to illustrate the history of nursing science in a recent historic review of nursing curriculum development (Ellis, 1982). In a retrospective study of nursing texts and journals from 1964 to 1974, Carper found that health was one of five key or representative concepts defined in the nursing curriculum. The other four were human beings (which included environment), nursing, patient/client, and behavior (Ellis, 1982). Donaldson and Crowley's analysis of the "structure of the discipline of nursing provides support for the four concepts as major ones in a knowledge structure or system of nursing" (Ellis, 1982, p. 410). There is agreement within nursing that nurses and their clients are in relationships concerned with health or health problems.

Concept Definitions

HUMAN BEINGS

Fawcett (1980) noted that the nursing theorists' conceptualizations of human beings view the person as a "biopsychosocial being who interacts with family members, the community, and other groups, as well as with the physical environment" (Fawcett, 1980, p. 11). However, each theorist presents her conceptualization of persons/human beings/society in "different and unique ways such as adaptive systems, behavioral subsystems or complementary four-dimensional energy fields" (Fawcett, 1980, p. 11). Regardless of how human beings are conceptualized by the theorists, nursing faculty will probably find its definitions including the statement of the client/person as a "biopsychosocial being who interacts with family members, the community, and other groups, as well as with the physical environment" (Fawcett, 1980, p. 11). This definition may be sufficient or may need to be elaborated upon and embellished, depending upon faculty's comfort level (Fig. 7).

ENVIRONMENT

When Nightingale described environment, she usually included only physical surroundings. Environment described in current curricula normally includes psychological, social or cultural elements in a full meaning of environment (Ellis, 1982). Environment might also be considered as the contextual space in which nursing is called for, initiated, and carried out (Ellis, 1982) (Fig. 8).

Definitions:	Bio-psycho-social being
	Individual-family (group)-community
	Interactive
	Adaptive system
	Behavioral system
	Four-dimensional energy field

Figure 7. Definitions of human beings.

Definitions:	Physical surroundings
	Physical, psychological, social, cultural surroundings
	Contextual space

Figure 8. Definitions of environment.

NURSING

Ellis (1982), in a historic review of conceptual frameworks, reports that "Nightingale conceptualized nursing as a science of health and described nursing . . . as primarily directed toward improving and managing the physical environment so that nature could heal the patient" (Ellis, 1982, p. 406). Ellis suggests that now there are two mainstreams of thought defining nursing: "(1) the care of the sick and (2) the promotion of health" (Ellis, 1982, p. 406).

Henderson's definition of nursing was a major shift from the task–procedure (care of the sick) perspective and one of the earliest, widely used definitions to present a conceptualization of nursing that included the ideas of function (process) and goal (Ellis, 1982). Henderson's definition of nursing was "to assist the individual, sick or well, in the performance of those activities contributing to health or its recovery (or to a peaceful death) that he would perform unaided if he had the necessary strength, will or knowledge. And to do this in such a way as to help him gain independence as rapidly as possible" (Ellis, 1982, p. 407). Ellis states Henderson's conceptualization was widely accepted by the nursing profession in the 1950s and 1960s and since the 1970s was extended with conceptualizations of nursing by Rogers, King, Orem, Roy, Johnson, Schlotfeldt, and others.

Wu (1979) contends that nursing has been primarily defined as a process with goals of nursing inherent in the process. Nursing has been viewed as an interpersonal process (Orlando and Travelbee), as a supporting process for human development (Erickson and Havinghurst), as an assisting process to individuals in the performance of those activities contributing to health or its recovery (Henderson), as a problem-solving process (Abdella), as a supporting process to the adaptation process (Roy and Neuman), as a behavioral process (Johnson), and as a health care process (Schlotfeldt).

Ellis (1982), in reviewing many conceptual frameworks found that nursing was often defined not as a process but in many instances only in terms of nursing goals: equilibrium, adaptation, repatterning, health, and self-care or enhancement of the self-care agency. To be complete and to follow the way in which nursing scholars and theorists are defining

Definitions:	The care of the sick and the promotion of health. Assist individual toward independent health, recovery or peaceful death.	
	A process:	Interpersonal
		Supporting
		Assisting
		Problem solving
		Adaptation
		Behavioral
		Health care
	Goal directed:	Equilibrium
		Adaptation
		Repatterning
		Health
		Self-care
		Health restoration
		Health maintenance
		Health promotion

Figure 9. Definitions of nursing.

nursing, faculty members now are finding that they are including both processes and goals of nursing in their definitions of nursing (Fig. 9).

HEALTH

Ellis (1982) states that in the past, descriptions of health in conceptual frameworks of nursing programs have been more disease centered than based on the promotion of health. She suggests that Smith's definition may be of help to faculty in developing health definitions.

> Smith has provided a useful resolution to the seemingly unrelated, multiple, and ambiguous views of health. These are (1) the clinical model based on the absence of signs and symptoms of disease, (2) the role performance model wherein adequate role performance is the common sense criteria of health, (3) the adaptive model in which health is a condition of effective interaction with one's physical and social environment, and (4) the

Definitions: Absence of signs and symptoms of disease

Adequate role performance

Effective interaction with one's physical and social environment

General sense of well-being

On a continuum

Figure 10. Definitions of health.

eudianomistic model that extends the meaning of health to general well-being and self-realization (Ellis, 1982, p. 408).

Fawcett (1980) states that models of most of the nursing theorists provide a definition of health by describing both the well and the ill person and environments conducive or detrimental to health. Obviously "an absence of illness or disease" is no longer sufficient for a definition of health. The possible definitions appropriate to curricular framework development are many and varied as well as ranging from simple definitions to complex definitions (Fig. 10).

LEARNER

The learner is often viewed as a cognitive, affective, and psychomotor being and therefore as a learner in all three domains (Bloom, 1956; Bruner, 1966; Gagné, 1974; Krathwohl, Bloom, and Masia, 1956; Skinner, 1968). The learner can also be described in relation to the teacher as dependent, independent, and interdependent, or as observer, participant, and practitioner (O'Kelley and McKinney, 1971) (Fig. 11).

Definitions: A cognitive, affective and psychomotor being in stages and processes of learning

Developmental

Dependent-independent-interdependent

Observer-participant-practitioner

Figure 11. Definitions of learner.

STRUCTURE

The structure of the conceptual framework is an organizational approach for the curriculum. It is a statement that relates the concepts and then provides definitions for the concepts. In a study, Quiring and Gray (1982) found that, historically, the organizational approaches used in curriculum have reflected at least six patterns: (1) subject matter, (2) core, (3) principles, (4) behavioral systems, (5) concepts, and (6) nursing models. The study was conducted for the purpose of identifying models employed to organize curricula and to estimate their frequency of use. Selected 4-year programs were surveyed to identify some of the ways they approached curriculum organization. Sixty-one percent of the 144 samples responded. Three questions were asked:

1. What method of program organization would be most characteristic of your school's undergraduate program?

   The overwhelming majority of schools attempted to integrate curriculum components through the use of some combination of concepts, threads, and the nursing process. Concepts were the major choice for a curriculum organization approach because they serve to unify or interrelate details.
2. Indicate the number of courses which used the organizing approach selected.

   The answers indicated that all the courses were involved.
3. Give one or more examples to further describe the methods of curriculum organization described.

   Man (human beings), health, and nursing were the major concepts for curricular organization with nursing process and the illness–wellness continuum as subconcepts of nursing and health.

Criteria for Evaluating Conceptual Framework

After the faculty members have defined human beings/society, health, nursing, and any other major concept, and have related the concepts to each other, the resulting framework or conceptual statement with definitions, if operational and intact, should answer six questions (Peterson, 1977):

1. Is nursing described?
2. Is the goal of nursing described?
3. Is why a client needs nursing described?
4. Is the nurse described?

5. Is the client described?
6. Is the context of nursing described?

Peterson (1977) further suggests criteria to determine if the conceptual framework is operational within the curriculum:

1. Do curricular materials indicate that a conceptual framework has guided the basic structure of the curriculum? (Objectives, threads, course titles.)
2. Is the terminology throughout the curriculum consistent with the conceptual framework?
3. Is there an agreed upon process of nursing that is consistent throughout the curriculum?
4. Can all faculty members describe the conceptual framework and is it evident in their teaching?
5. Do all the students' written assignments reflect the conceptual framework?
6. Do clinical assignments, care plans reflect the conceptual framework? Is the students' view of the patient consistent with the conceptual framework?
7. Can students describe the conceptual framework and how they personally use it?

FUNCTION

Sequence of Content

Wu (1979) suggests that once a conceptual framework for a nursing program is agreed upon, the task is to identify the major elements of the concepts that will appear and reappear at each level of the curriculum and thus provide elements for the content organization and sequence in the curriculum. The concepts are subjected to a process whereby range of scope and levels of complexity are delineated. The number of persons in a relationship (person, dyad-family, community) and chronology (developmental stages) are examples of possible elements or subconcepts of human beings; range of cues (simple to complex) and history (familiar to unfamiliar; common and frequent to unusual and nonrecurring events) may be concepts of learning. Noncomplicated to complicated conditions, stable and predictable to unstable unpredictable events or conditions, healthy to unhealthy conditions may be the elements of health; concrete to abstract reasoning may be one organizational element for nursing (Table 8).

TABLE 8. ELEMENTS OF CONCEPTS THAT AID IN THEIR SEQUENCING

Concept	Elements (Subconcepts) to Aid Sequencing of Content
Persons	Number in a relationship
	Person, dyad-family, community
	Chronology
	Developmental stages
Learning	Range of cues
	Simple to complex
	History
	Familiar to unfamiliar
	Common, frequent to unusual and nonrecurring events
Health	Noncomplicated to complicated
	Stable and predictable to unstable, unpredictable
	Healthy to unhealthy
Nursing	Concrete to abstract reasoning

Posner (1976) presents questions for faculty consideration when determining the content sequences in the curriculum:

1. What are the relationships between the concepts about what the student is to learn and in what sequence can the content be ordered so that the organization is consistent with those relationships? In other words, are not only the concepts ordered in sequence, but their relationships and interrelationships (the conceptual framework) throughout the curriculum (Fig. 12)?
2. What are the conceptual properties (attributes) of the concepts to be learned and in what sequence can content be ordered so that it is logically consistent in organization to the attributes of the concepts? If the concept of personhood/society is defined as having individual, family/groups, community as its attributes, are these attributes reflected sequentially in the curriculum for the provision of a logically consistent organization and developmental progression of the concept for student acquisition and understanding (Fig. 13)?
3. How are concepts in the curriculum and their relationships developed and in what ways can they be ordered in a sequence? Is there a sequential progression of the relational attributes and characteristics of the concepts? Are the relational aspects of the conceptual framework ordered in a sequence? The concepts of the conceptual framework are not only related and ordered in a progressive sequence but their attribute's relationships are as well (Fig. 14).

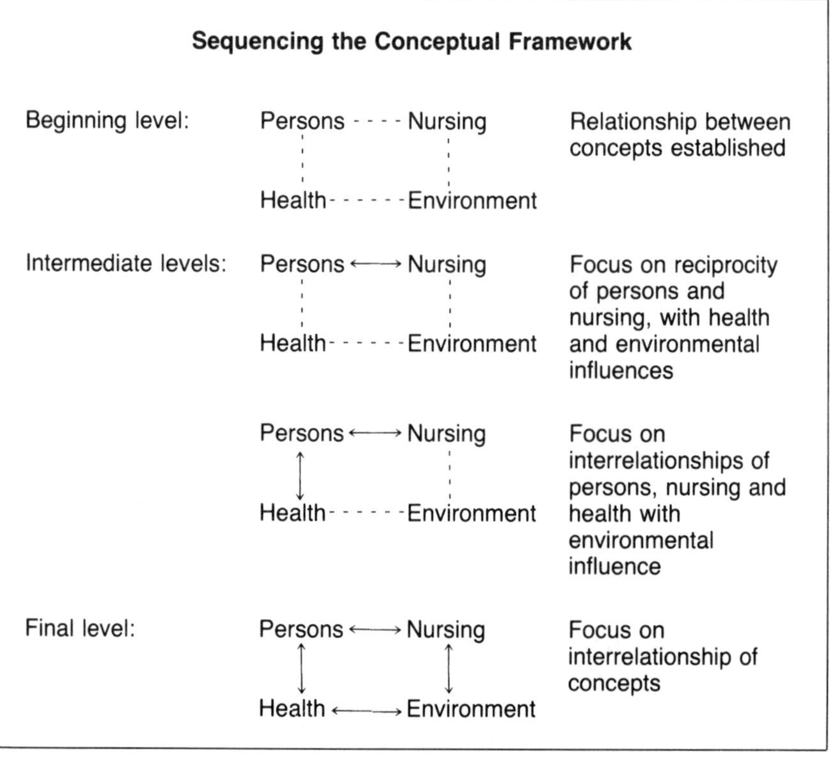

Figure 12. Sequencing of the relationship of the concepts of persons, nursing, health, and environment.

Concept Sequencing via Attributes

Beginning level:	Concept of personhood established (individual-family-community)
Intermediate levels:	Focus on individual Focus on family and groups
Final level:	Focus on community

Figure 13. Sequencing of the subconcepts of the concept personhood.

Sequencing Related to Subconcepts' Relationships

Beginning level: Persons-nursing-health-environment relationship established; attributes (subconcepts) of each developed.

Concept	*Subconcepts*
Persons:	Individual, family, community
Nursing:	Goal directed toward restoration, maintenance and/or promotion
Health:	On a continuum
Environment:	Controlled, uncontrolled

Intermediate levels: Relationship of individual and the nursing goal of health restoration in a controlled environment developed

Relationship of family and/or groups and the nursing goal of health maintenance in a less controlled environment developed

Final level: Relationship of community and the nursing goal of health promotion in a rather open and less confining environment developed

Figure 14. Sequencing of the relationships of the concepts and the relationships of the concepts' subconcepts.

4. How does the student learn and in what sequence can the content be patterned so that it is consistent with the learning process? Aspects to be considered when determining the sequence of content for student learning are: What are the prerequisites needed? How familiar is the student with the content? What is the past experience of the student related to the content? How difficult is the content? What is the interest of the student in the content? What value is desired to become internalized by the student? Where is the student developmentally (Fig. 15)?
5. How will the student use the content after she or he has learned it and in what sequence can the content be ordered so that it is consistent with her or his usage of it? Are content and skills presented in the beginning of the curriculum used and needed in the rest of the nursing program? What is the reason for pre-

Learning Process Considerations for Sequencing Content

Prerequisites

Familiarity

Past experiences

Difficulty level

Value internalization

Interest

Growth and development

Figure 15. Considerations in the learning process.

senting certain content in the beginning, middle, and end of the curriculum? The answer to these questions is the utilization value of the contents (Fig. 16).

Posner (1976) identified several possible conceptual sequences for content from which the faculty may choose in answering the five questions that it asks when determining in what order to sequence the content. The sequences can be categorized into two distinct "regions." One region is the subject matter region which includes world-related sequences and concept-related sequences. The second region is the learner region which includes two considerations for the ordering of content: the learning process and the utilization or usage process.

SUBJECT MATTER REGION

World-Related Sequences. One type of sequence, world-related, includes sequences of content related to *space*, *time*, and *physical* attributes. Content sequences related to *space* would be having learning experiences that start in a controlled-closed system such as a hospital, then moving into clinics, and finally into the community where spatially the experiences are more wide ranging and independent than in the hospital.

Examples of *time* sequences would be anything chronologic, such as growth and development, as a curricular organizer. Organizing by *physical* attributes could be arranging a curriculum by biologic systems: musculoskeletal, gastrointestinal–biliary, cardiovascular–respiratory, and reproductive (Fig. 17).

Content Presented Based on Utilization Value

Beginning level:	Introduction to intramuscular and subcutaneous injections
Intermediate and final levels:	Frequent performance of intramuscular and subcutaneous injections

Figure 16. Sequencing related to predicted frequency of use.

Concept-Related Sequences. Another type of sequence available for faculty's consideration, concept-related, reflects the organization of the conceptual, more abstract words. *Class-related, propositional-related, sophistication of propositional-related,* and *logical prerequisites* are types of this kind of sequence.

CLASS-RELATED. Class-related sequences refer to the progressive development of the properties or attributes of a concept (class) identified by

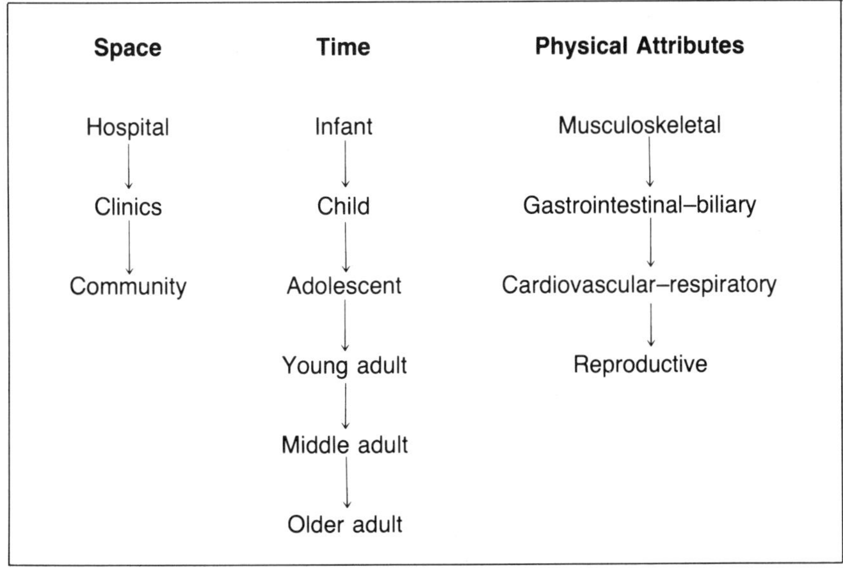

Figure 17. World-related sequences of space, time, and physical attributes.

the faculty. If one of the attributes of nursing defined was the set of goals of restoration, maintenance, and promotion, then these goals of nursing would be the nursing theme of the curriculum and the sequences of content would follow that theme.

PROPOSITIONAL-RELATED. Propositional-related sequences use relationships such as a conceptual framework, a theory or model on which to base the curriculum. When a conceptual framework is operational, the relationship of the concepts to each other as well as the relationships that form from the framework determine the sequence of content and learning activities in the curriculum.

SOPHISTICATION OF PROPOSITONAL-RELATED. Sophistication of propositional-related sequences recognize that levels of sophistication are found in the conceptual framework and thus are concerned with presenting the concrete before the abstract or the simple before the complex. Propositional sophistication-related sequences are most obviously found when an existing model of nursing is used, such as Orem's model of self-care or Roy's adaptation model, where the paradigm is at first simply presented, then progressively developed so that by the time of graduation, the graduate is a model of the model.

LOGICAL PREREQUISITE. The use of logical prerequisite sequences is simply organizing the curriculum according to some logical progression. If the faculty thinks the concept of personhood is defined by the attributes of individual, group, and community, then the progression in the organization scheme is individual before group before community (Fig. 18).

LEARNER REGION

Learning Process Sequences. Learning process sequences draw primarily on knowledge about the psychology and process of learning as a basis for curriculum development and instructional planning. Included in learning process sequences are the topics of the *empiric prerequisites, content difficulty, learner interest, learner development,* and *value internalization.*

EMPIRIC PREREQUISITE SEQUENCES. Empiric prerequisite sequences take place when the learning of one skill facilitates or makes possible the learning of a subsequent skill. For example, the skill of sterile and clean technique is most often included early in the curriculum before subsequent techniques and procedures requiring its use are presented. The whole idea of having a "skills course" in the beginning of the curriculum is based on the principle of the empiric prerequisite sequence.

LEVEL OF DIFFICULTY SEQUENCES. Sequences by level of difficulty simply place the less difficult before the more difficult content in the curriculum. Problems arise when faculty disagrees as to what is more difficult or less difficult. The placement of content related to nursing of the childbearing family is a good example. Some place the content (totally) in the beginning of the curriculum, others in the middle, and still others as a senior learning activity. Which is right as far as difficulty level is concerned? If the content were integrated within a framework other than the subject matter framework, it would be in all levels, but in increasing levels of difficulty.

LEARNER INTEREST SEQUENCES. Sequences related to learner interest involve organizing content that is intrinsically interesting and in which the learner has had some limited experience, but that still remains a challenge. One might contend that the nursing curriculum has traditionally been organized in an interest sequence with the eagerly awaited fundamentals of nursing course followed first by the medical–surgical, hospital activities. Students want to perform procedures and nursing fundamentals provide this opportunity, as does medical–surgical hospital nursing; thus student interest can be and has been used (maybe unbeknown to faculty) as a curriculum organizer. The broad health-related, community content is reserved for last because when interest is less hospital-oriented and sick-centered, the student is ready to focus on other aspects of nursing, in particular, illness prevention and health promotion.

LEARNER DEVELOPMENT SEQUENCES. Sequences that take into account learner growth and development deal with changes in the learner that occur as a result of the maturation process, both professional and personal. For curriculum sequences relative to the maturation level, decisions must be made as to what requires more maturity in a given situation or context. For example, does care of one hospitalized individual or the utilization of resources in the community for the health care of family and groups require more maturity? The answer may seem obvious, but it could be argued either way.

VALUE INTERNALIZATION SEQUENCES. Sequences of value internalization aim to have the student internalize an attitude or value, usually within the Krathwohl, Bloom, and Masia's (1956) taxonomy of value receiving, re-

Concept-Related Sequences

Class-Related

Concept (Class): Nursing

Attributes:

Nursing goals	Roles
Restoration of health	Wholly compensatory
Maintenance of health	Partially compensatory
Promotion of health	Educative supportive

Propositional-Related

Proposition:

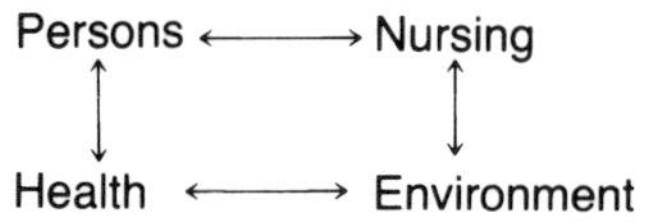

Persons ⟷ Nursing
↕ ↕
Health ⟷ Environment

Proposition development:

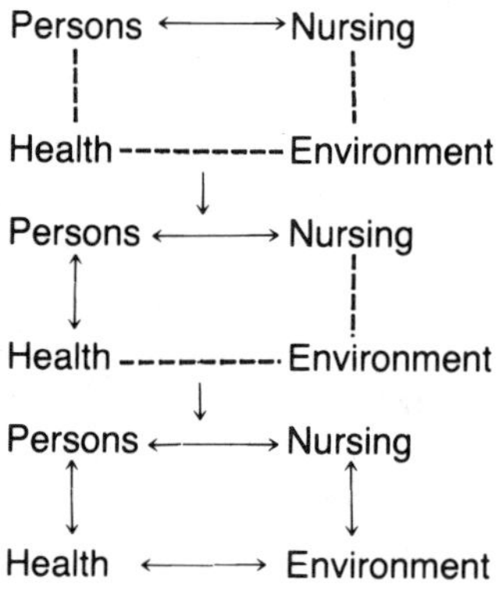

Persons ⟷ Nursing
¦ ¦
Health --------- Environment
↓
Persons ⟷ Nursing
↕ ¦
Health --------- Environment
↓
Persons ⟷ Nursing
↕ ↕
Health ⟷ Environment

Propositional Sophistication-Related

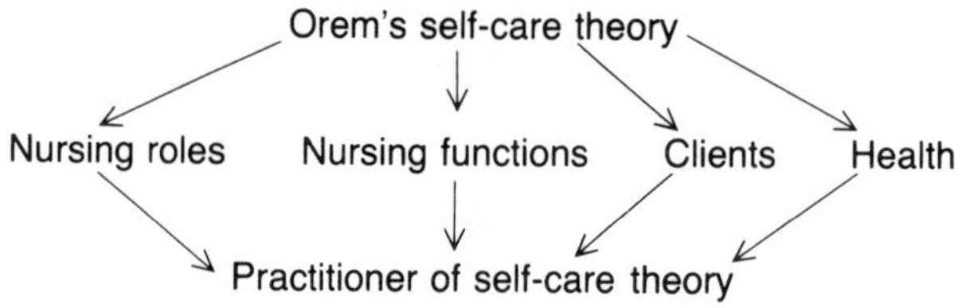

Orem's self-care theory
↓
Nursing roles — Nursing functions — Clients — Health
↓
Practitioner of self-care theory

cont.

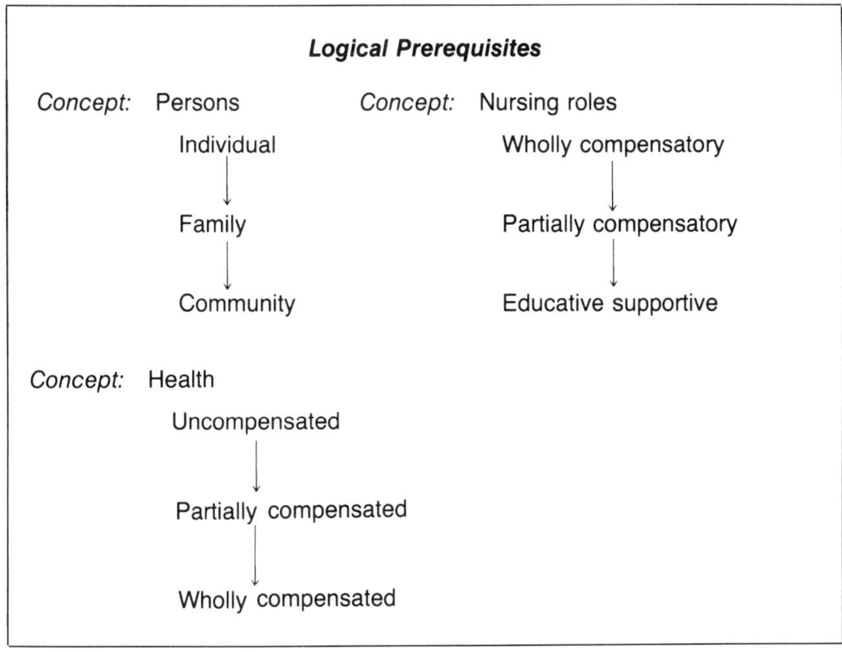

Figure 18. Conceptual curricular organization by class, proposition, propositional sophistication, and logical prerequisites.

sponding, valuing, organizing, and characterization. The socialization of the student into the nursing profession is an example of this. Until the present, socialization as a value sequence has been little used as evidenced by the fact that a senior level trends or issues course was the extent of the experience a student had in preparation for socialization into the profession. Now in some curricula, basic concept and nursing issues are taught in the beginning of the curriculum, and oftentimes as a separate course. Faculty has planned socialization activity sequences throughout the curriculum to the point that in the senior year, the internalization of the value, socialization into the profession, is realized (Fig. 19).

Utilization Sequences. Three contexts are considered in sequences related to utilization: *social, personal,* and *career*. Units of study are organized on the basis of the knowledge and skills needed to perform in an occupation or career with little regard to personal and social devel-

Learning Process Sequences

Empiric Prerequisite

Beginning level:	*Prerequisite skill:*	Sterile/clean technique
Intermediate, final and graduate levels:	*Subsequent skills:*	Catheterization Tracheostomy care Dressing change Clean-catch U.A. Suture set-up Injections Intravenous therapy

Level of Difficulty

Childbearing Family

Focus: Mostly controlled variables	Labor & delivery— health restoration
Focus: More or less controlled variables	Prenatal— health maintenance
Focus: Complex and many unpredictable variables	Postnatal— health promotion

Learner Interest

Beginning level:	SKILLS
Intermediate levels:	SKILLS—HOSPITAL
	HOSPITAL—Clinics—Community
Final level:	Hospital—CLINICS—COMMUNITY

Learner Development

Beginning level: Observer	*Beginning level:* Health care environment with few variables
Intermediate level: Observer-participant	*Intermediate level:* Health care environment with many variables
Final level: Participant; Quasi-practitioner	*Final level:* Health care environment with complex variables

cont.

	Value Internalization
Value:	Socialization
Beginning level:	Introduction to nursing concepts, trends and issues
Intermediate levels:	Concepts, trends, issues integrated
Final level:	Trends, issues facing the beginning practitioner

Figure 19. Sequencing the process of learning related to prerequisites, learner interest, development, and internalization of values.

opment in schools with minimal liberal studies. In nursing programs situated in universities whose mission is to produce the liberally educated person, however, social and personal aspects are prominently considered along with career concerns.

The two subtypes of utilization-related sequences are *procedure* (process) sequences and *anticipated frequency of utilization* sequences.

PROCESS SEQUENCES. An example of process sequences related to utilization value in the curriculum is the use of the nursing process or decision making as a curricular organizer. Since decision making and the nursing process, for that matter, can be utilized in social, personal, and career contexts, they are natural organizers for a nursing curriculum. This does not mean that one step of decision making is learned in one year and another in the next. It does mean that decision making in social, personal, and career (discipline) contexts is taught early in the beginning content and skills and threaded by planned sequences throughout the curriculum. As the understanding, appreciation, and development of the social, personal, and career contexts develop, the complexity of decision-making skills increases.

ANTICIPATED FREQUENCY SEQUENCES. Anticipated frequency of utilization is the principle employed when the order of the phenomena taught is based on the anticipated frequency of utilization in the students' future experience and activities. Skills and interpersonal laboratories placed in the beginning of a curriculum are positioned there according to this principle. Throughout the curriculum and in practice, certain skills will be needed and therefore will be taught first (Fig. 20).

Utilization Sequences

Process

Beginning level:	Introduction of nursing process/decision-making skills
Intermediate levels:	Utilization of nursing process/decision-making skills in hospital
	Utilization of nursing process/decision-making skills in hospital, clinic
Final level:	Utilization of nursing process/decision-making skills in hospital, clinic, community, and personal and professional goals

Anticipated Frequency

Beginning level:	Intramuscular injection in learning laboratory
Intermediate levels:	Intramuscular injection in hospital, clinics
	Intramuscular injection in hospital, clinics, community
Final level:	Intramuscular injection as practitioner
Beginning level:	Interpersonal relationship skills in learning laboratory
Intermediate levels:	Interpersonal relationship skills with individuals
	Interpersonal relationship skills with families and groups
Final level:	Interpersonal relationship skills with community resources

Figure 20. Sequencing related to the usage of a process and frequency of usage.

CONTINUITY OF CONTENT

As the framework provides a means of organization and ordering by way of sequences of concepts and elements within the concepts, it also provides a means for content and learning continuity by providing threading elements throughout the curriculum. Continuity as an organizer is provided by the reiteration of the major curricular elements, thereby providing recurring emphasis for the learner and teacher (Tyler, 1950).

Continuity

Beginning level:	Research, teaching, leadership, nursing process introduced
Intermediate levels:	Research, teaching, leadership, nursing process integrated in courses
Final level:	Research, teaching, leadership, nursing process synthesized and conceptualized by graduate as nursing process

Figure 21. Continuity: reiteration of research, teaching, leadership, and nursing process.

Common continuity organizers are research, leadership, nursing process, and teaching. If organizer elements are found in all courses, continuity is provided throughout the curriculum (Fig. 21).

INTEGRATION OF CONTENT

The process of integration occurs in the curriculum as organizing elements become unified within the learner. Wu (1979) states that the purpose of integration is to unify all of the curricular elements (those for sequencing and those for continuity) so that they appear connected rather than as separate unrelated parts. Integration occurs as content is fused and synthesized within an organizational framework of the curriculum.

Continuity, sequence, and integration were lacking in the traditional "subject matter" curriculum model which did not have the organizing elements of a conceptual framework. Students under this model achieved compartmentalized learning with little or no concept of how each component of the curriculum related to the other components. Integration is achieved in the learner by bringing together content and subject matter through organizing elements, threads, and sequences of the major concepts. The result is a unified curriculum and a unified concept of the discipline in which and with which the student will learn, the teacher will teach, and the graduate will practice.

Organization is the key to a logical curriculum. With a review of Wu (1979) and Posner (1976), faculty will find there are many possible ways of organizing the curriculum. The major decisions will be to decide in which way and with what elements.

REFERENCES

Ausubel, D. P. *Educational Psychology: A Cognitive View*. New York: Holt, Rinehart and Winston, 1968.

Bartlett, F. C. *Remembering*. Cambridge, England: Cambridge University Press, 1932.

Bloom, B. S. (Ed.). *Taxonomy of Educational Objectives, the Classification of Educational Goals, Handbook I: Cognitive Domain*. New York: David McKay, 1956.

Bruner, J. S. *Toward a Theory of Instruction*. Cambridge: Belknap Press of Harvard University Press, 1966.

Ellis, R. Conceptual issues in nursing. *Nurs Outlook,* 1982, 30, 406–410.

Fawcett, J. A framework for analysis and evaluation of conceptual models of nursing. *Nurse Educator,* 1980, 5, 10–14.

Gagné, R. M. *Essentials of Learning for Instruction*. Hinsdale, Illinois: Dryden Press, 1974.

Hall, K. B. Current trends in the use of conceptual frameworks in nursing education. *J Nurs Educ,* 1979, 18, 26–29.

Huckabay, L. M. D. *Conditions of Learning and Instruction in Nursing: Modularized*. St. Louis: C. V. Mosby, 1980.

Krathwohl, D. R., Bloom, B. S., & Masia, B. B. *Taxonomy of Educational Goals, Handbook II: Affective Domain*. New York: David McKay, 1956.

O'Kelley, L. E., & McKinney, G. A conceptual model for medical-surgical nursing. *Nurs Outlook*, 1971, 19, 731–736.

Peterson, C. Questions frequently asked about the development of a conceptual framework. *J Nurs Educ,* 1977, 16, 22–32.

Posner, G., & Strike, K. A. A categorization scheme for principles of sequencing content. *Rev Educ Research,* 1976, 46, 665–690.

Quiring, J., & Gray, G. Organizing approaches used in curriculum design. *J Nurs Educ,* 1982, 21, 38–44.

Skinner, B. F. *The Technology of Teaching*. Englewood Cliffs, N.J.: Prentice-Hall, 1968.

Tyler, R. W. *Basic Principles of Curriculum and Instruction*. Chicago: The University of Chicago, 1950.

Wu, R. R. Designing a curriculum model. *J Nurs Educ,* 1979, 18, 13–21.

4

Curricular Objectives

Along with the philosophy and conceptual framework, behavioral objectives or outcomes expected of the graduate serve as guides for curricular development and revision.

DEVELOPMENT

There are several areas of consideration faculty must take into account when determining what objectives should be attained by the graduate of its program.

One document for faculty to consider in determining the behavioral objectives is the state's nurse practice act. The nurse practice act provides competencies and behaviors expected of registered nurses which must be considered in their educational preparation. Another consideration is the behaviors tested in the National Council Licensure Examination (NCLEX)—also known as the state board examination. The examination focuses on the nursing process with the behaviors of assessing, planning, implementing, and evaluating patient/client situations (McCarty, 1982; Smeltzer, 1982). The National League for Nursing (NLN) has delineated competencies and characteristics for the associate degree graduate and baccalaureate degree graduate, which faculty may very well want to review before writing the objectives of the program (National League for Nursing, 1979, 1982). A related guideline would be the American Nurses Association (ANA) Standards of Practice (Standards: Nursing Practice, 1973). Some programs simply use the ANA Standards of Practice as the objectives of their program.

Another very important source is the profession's, in particular the practicing profession's (nursing service), expectations of graduates coming into practice. Sullivan and Brye (1983) suggest the Delphi technique as a tool that can be utilized for obtaining such survey-type information from the profession. The Delphi technique is "intended to survey the 'expert' opinion of persons knowledgeable in a particular field of study" (Sullivan and Brye, 1983, p. 187). It is a

> tool utilizing sequential questionnaires sent to experts in a particular field who respond . . . to the . . . probability of future events occurring in the profession. The participants receive feedback in the form of the consensus of their peers following each round of questionnaires . . . This process tends to produce group consensus of evolving trends. The resulting decisions of the respondents can form a base of information that can be used to examine projected curriculum goals (Sullivan and Brye, 1983, pp. 187–188).

Also a consideration in determining the objectives of the program are the concept definitions set forth by faculty and the resultant organizational framework of the curriculum. The concepts are reflected in the outcomes of the graduate since they are the basis for the curriculum content and experiences. It may be remembered also that one of the criteria for determining an operational conceptual framework is that the concepts are reflected in the outcomes of the program (Peterson, 1977).

STRUCTURE

Subject Matter

Three areas of content or subject matter are prominent in the objectives of most nursing programs: role, responsibility, and performance (Quiring and Gray, 1979). Kramer (1981) suggests that the baccalaureate nurse roles are care-giving, management, health promotion and supervision, teaching and counseling, and health and illness screening. The associate degree graduate attains the role of the care-giver (Fig. 22).

The behaviors of responsibility are usually seen in relation to the graduate's acceptance of responsibility for her actions and for continued learning. Performance objectives are generally in the form of or related to the graduate's use of the nursing process as a member of the health care team (Fig. 23).

Behavior

The cognitive domain (Bloom, 1956) and affective domain (Krathwohl et al., 1956) taxonomies of behavior are commonly used by nursing faculty in writing behavioral objectives. Most, but not all, of the behaviors expected of the graduate are at the application cognitive level and the receptive or valuing affective level. Since NCLEX primarily tests behaviors of the nurse at the application level, credence is given to

Baccalaureate Graduate

Upon completion of the nursing program, the graduate will perform caregiving, management, health promotion and supervision, teaching and counseling, and health and illness screening based in a framework of self-care.

Associate Graduate

Upon completion of the nursing program, the graduate will perform caregiving based in a framework of adaptation.

Figure 22. Behavioral objectives of those graduating from baccalaureate and associate programs according to Kramer (1981).

application being the minimal level of behaviors for the graduate of a nursing program.

The expected behavior may be written in a typical behavioral objective style (one subject, one verb, one condition) (Gronlund, 1978; Reilly, 1980)(Fig. 24), or in a competency statement (a statement including more than one behavior with accompanying enabling objectives (Guineé, 1978) (Fig. 25). Whatever the case, the terminal behavior is visible to the graduate, faculty, and consumer; it is a guideline for instruction and evaluation for learning and for determining the competencies of the graduate.

Responsibility

Upon completion of the nursing program, the graduate will accept responsibility for continual professional growth and development.

Performance

Upon completion of the nursing program, the graduate will use the nursing process based in a conservation framework in all areas of health care.

Figure 23. Behavioral objectives related to responsibility and performance.

The graduate of an associate program in nursing will perform as a manager of nursing care for a group of clients with common, well-defined health problems in structured settings.

Figure 24. Behavioral objective.

FUNCTION

Outcomes put the philosophy and conceptual framework in behavioral terms, necessary to be attained if the student is to graduate, just as outcomes for a course are necessary to attain if the student is to promote from course to course.

The function of the behavioral objectives is to provide guidelines for faculty members in determining learning activities for the students in order for them to attain the objectives of the curriculum. Additional functions are that they provide the behaviors for student evaluation as well as faculty and course evaluation.

Behaviors Attained

According to Joyce and Weil (1980), there are four categories of behaviors from which the faculty may choose to write the behavioral objectives expected of the graduate: conditioned behavior, information-processing behavior, social interaction behavior, and personal awareness.

As a manager of nursing care for a group of clients with common, well-defined health problems in structured settings, the associate degree nursing graduate:

- Assesses and sets nursing care priorities.
- With guidance, provides client care utilizing resources and other nursing personnel commensurate with their educational preparation and experience.
- Seeks guidance to assist other nursing personnel to develop skills in giving nursing care.

Figure 25. Competency statement (Competencies of the Associate Degree nurse on entry into practice). *(Adapted from Nurs Outlook, 24:457, 1978.).*

At the completion of the program, the graduate will perform accurately techniques and skills necessary in the health care environment.

At the completion of the skills laboratory, the student will be able to correctly, quickly and with minimal effort insert a nasogastic (NG) tube.

Figure 26. Behavioral objectives expected of conditioned behavior.

CONDITIONED BEHAVIOR

The world or the environment is the medium for conditioned learning. The "environment" may be an instructor, written materials, video tape or role models. Mimic behavior is the outcome of conditioning. The performance or behaviors expected of conditioning are mastery, convergence, programmed, modeling, and reconstruction. Psychomotor skills and memorized lists are examples of learned conditioned behavior. A metaphor for conditioning is that the student represents a mechanical mirror in that the student is a mirror (mimic) of that which was learned. The learning is "mechanical" in that it is a conditioned, not reasoned, behavior. The learner is not to waver or deviate from the knowledge or steps of a process or skill, but to repeat it or mimic what has been learned.

Conditioned behavior is a legitimate behavior to be attained in a nursing program. It generally is not seen as a terminal behavior, but is indeed in the objectives of lessons, units, and some basic courses. Although often not written as a terminal objective, it is seen as an enabling behavior to the final outcomes of the program (Fig. 26).

INFORMATION-PROCESSING BEHAVIOR

The mind is the medium for learning in information processing with outcomes of creative, critical, and free thinking. The kind of performances to be expected of information-processing learning are dependent upon the student's stage of cognitive processing. Bruner (1966) suggests that there are three levels of information processing: enactive, iconic, and symbolic; Piaget (Gallagher, 1974) suggests three also: sensorimotor, concrete, and symbolic.

At the enactive and sensorimotor level, the behavior is that of recognizing or understanding something by what it does or how it behaves. Reasoning is not a large part of the first stage; recognition is.

If the student is at the iconic or concrete stage of learning, once again reasoning is only a limited part of the behavior. Imagery, and to some degree conceptualization, is the outcome of iconic learning, but again it is limited in breadth.

Application:	At the conclusion of N104, Nursing in the Childbearing Family, the student will be able to apply the nursing process within the framework of the childbearing family.
Analysis:	At the conclusion of N410, Nursing Issues, the student will be able to analyze issues in nursing as influenced by economic, political, social, and professional factors.
Synthesis:	Before performing patient care in the clinical setting in N301, Critical Care Nursing, the student will develop a plan of care based on the nursing diagnosis.
Evaluation:	At the conclusion of N402, Nursing Research, the student will be able to critically review research in relation to its problem, design, and findings for the purpose of its utilization value in the health care setting.

Figure 27. Information-processing behavioral objectives framed in Bloom's (1956) taxonomy of cognitive behaviors.

At the symbolic or abstract thinking level, behavioral expectations are critical thinking, reactive thinking, analysis, problem solving, evaluation and synthesis, divergence, and origination. The learner is an organic lamp in the information-processing metaphor, as opposed to the mechanical mirror of conditioning. The performance is not imitative but idiosyncratic. The world is produced by the learner rather than mimicked. The category of information processing is the one most reflected in terminal objectives of nursing programs. Indeed the symbolic, abstract stage of information processing is what reaches the terminal objectives, but the preceding stages are very much a part of the learning process within the program and may even be found in some objectives of lessons or units, making them enabling objectives to the terminal ones (Fig. 27).

SOCIAL INTERACTION BEHAVIOR

The learning medium for social interaction learning is the self with others. Sensitivity to the dynamics of groups and social interaction are the outcomes. Performance to be expected and thus reflected in the behavioral objectives are leadership, group interaction, and group problem solving. In general what is to be expected is social or group problem solving and interpersonal and group skills (Fig. 28).

PERSONAL AWARENESS

The source of learning for personal awareness is the self, and therefore the outcome is self-awareness. Behaviors to be expected of the learner

Upon completion of this program, the graduate will interact with other members in the health care system for a positive impact on the health care for the consumer.

Figure 28. Behavioral objective expected from learning in social interaction.

After the completion of the program, the graduate will have developed a beginning ethic of practice that supports decisions made related to the client's health care.

Figure 29. Behavioral objective expected from personal awareness learning.

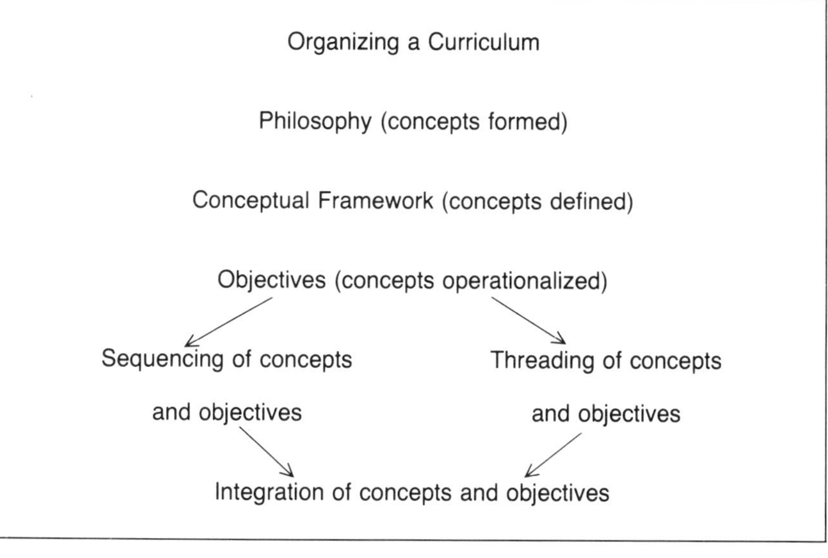

Figure 30. Curriculum organization.

include empathy, personal awareness, insightfulness, introspection, reflection, value clarification, self-responsibility, personal complexity, and flexibility. The behavioral objectives addressed in the responsibility role are a result of personal awareness learning activities (Fig. 29).

The function, therefore, of the objectives is to provide faculty with guidelines for learning activities and behavioral development throughout the curriculum. The terminal behavioral objectives are reflected in lessons, units, courses, and level objectives. The behaviors expected and developed by the students are of four categories: conditioning, information processing, social interaction, and personal awareness—all operationalizing the philosophy and conceptual framework throughout the curriculum (Fig. 30).

REFERENCES

Bloom, B. (Ed.). *Taxonomy of Educational Objectives, the Classification of Educational Goals, Handbook I: Cognitive Domain*. New York: David McKay, 1956.

Bruner, J. S. *Toward a Theory of Instruction*. Cambridge: Belknap of Harvard University Press, 1966.

Competencies of the Associate Degree nurse on entry into practice. *Nurs Outlook*, 1978, 24, 457–458.

Gallagher, J. M. The development of thinking according to Jean Piaget. In J. F. Adams (Ed.), *Understanding Adolescence*. Boston: Allyn and Bacon, 1974.

Gronlund, N. E. *Stating Objectives for Classroom Instruction* (2nd ed.). New York: Macmillan, 1978.

Guineé, K. *Teaching and Learning in Nursing*. New York: Macmillan, 1978.

Joyce, B., & Weil, M. *Models of Teaching* (2nd ed.). Englewood Cliffs, N.J.: Prentice-Hall, 1980.

Kramer, M. Philosophical foundations of baccalaureate nursing education. *Nurs Outlook*, 1981, 29, 224–228.

Krathwohl, D. R., Bloom, B. S., & Masia, B. B. *Taxonomy of Educational Objectives, the Classification of Educational Goals, Handbook II: Affective Domain*. New York: David McKay, 1956.

McCarty, P. New RN exam based on nursing process. *Amer Nurse*, March, 1982, pp. 1, 10, 28.

National League for Nursing. *Characteristics of Baccalaureate Education in Nursing*. New York: National League for Nursing Publication 15–1758, 1979.

National League for Nursing. *Competencies of Graduates of Nursing Programs*. New York: National League for Nursing Publication 14–1905, 1982.

Peterson, C. Questions frequently asked about the development of a conceptual framework. *J Nurs Educ*. 1977, 16, 22–32.

Quiring, J., & Gray, G. T. Is baccalaureate education based on a patchwork curriculum? *Nurs Outlook*, 1979, 27, 708–713.

Reilly, D. *Behavioral Objectives—Evaluation in Nursing* (2nd ed.). New York: Appleton-Century-Crofts, 1980.

Smeltzer, S. O. The new state board exam. *Nurs Outlook*, 1982, 30, 312–313.

Standards: Nursing Practice. Kansas City, Missouri: American Nurses Association, 1973.

Sullivan, E., & Brye, C. Nursing's future: Use of the Delphi technique for curriculum planning. *J Nurs Educ*, 1983, 22, 187–189.

5

Conclusion of Unit 1

AN EXAMPLE OF CONTEXT EVALUATION FOR PLANNING DECISIONS

Questions Asked for Data Gathering	*Sources of Data*
What is the institution's philosophy?	1. Catalog of institution: its reference to its philosophy and mission. (This will be one of the parameters of faculty's philosophy development.)
What are the nursing profession's beliefs?	1. Review of literature, especially ANA and NLN documents. (This will be one of the parameters of faculty's philosophy development.)
What is the philosophy of the faculty? What is the philosophy of each faculty member about human beings? Nursing? Health? Environment? The learner? Nursing education?	1. Survey of faculty 2. Pooling of survey results 3. Document of faculty's majority beliefs circulated to faculty for refinement 4. Small group discussion among faculty members of survey results 5. Results of small groups distributed to faculty for review and return

	6. Committee develops final document for review and refinement to be distributed to faculty for approval or further revision
What are the concepts basic to the nursing program?	1. Philosophy and beliefs of the nursing program 2. Outcomes of a curriculum development workshop for faculty or small group sessions
What does faculty believe about the concepts?	1. Philosophy of nursing program
What is faculty's skill in conceptualizing?	1. Conceptual framework workshop for assessment and practice in conceptualizing
What is faculty's understanding of a conceptual framework?	1. Conceptual framework workshop for assessment of faculty's understanding of conceptual frameworks 2. Small group discussion on what is a conceptual framework and its merits, or lack thereof
Is there one or more nursing theorist's conceptualizations faculty particularly likes?	1. Faculty survey 2. Faculty small group discussion 3. Pooling faculty's responses for distribution 4. Refining faculty's responses after first distribution and resubmitting to faculty either through memorandum or small group discussion
What are the common concepts in other programs and how are they developed and implemented?	1. Literature review of nursing journals 2. Numerous NLN publications 3. Survey of nursing programs

How does faculty define nursing? Persons? Health? Environment? The learner? Nursing education?	1. Survey of faculty 2. Pool data 3. Return results 4. Small group discussions 5. Committee develops general definitions for faculty review and faculty approval
Are Peterson's six questions answered in the conceptual framework?	1. Peterson (1977)
How should the concepts and learning process be sequenced? How should the curriculum be organized in a logically consistent manner? What should be the sequencing organizers? What should be the continuity organizers?	1. Identified concepts 2. Faculty definitions of concepts 3. Wu (1979), Posner (1976) 4. Faculty small group discussions to look at ways of sequencing and providing continuity 5. Survey of other programs to see how they sequence content and provide continuity 6. Sharing of information from small groups and surveys to faculty through documents or more small groups 7. Results of small groups distributed to faculty for review and return 8. Committee develops final document for review and refinement to be distributed to faculty for approval or further revision
What behaviors in the State's Nurse Practice Act are expected of the graduate?	1. State Nurse Practice Act

What are the behaviors expected for licensure	1. NCLEX reviews 2. Literature reviews about NCLEX 3. State board newsletters
What does the profession suggest as behaviors for the graduate?	1. NLN: Competencies of Graduates of Nursing Programs (Pub. No. 14-1905, 1982) 2. ANA Standards of Practice 3. Literature review in nursing journals
What expectations does the practicing profession have of the new graduate?	1. Outreach program where faculty and nursing service discuss curriculum development (predicted and current) and expectations of graduates, as well as students' behaviors
What is the framework of the expectations of the graduate?	1. Philosophy of program 2. Conceptual framework of the program
What expectations does the consumer have of the graduate?	1. Literature review 2. Consumer panel
What are the expectations of faculty of student and graduate behaviors?	1. Survey of faculty 2. Pooling results of faculty survey 3. Distributing results of pooling 4. Small group discussion among faculty members of survey results 5. Results of small groups distributed to faculty for review and return 6. Committee develops final document for review and refinement to be distributed to faculty for approval or further revision

PLANNING DECISIONS

With the data gathered for context evaluation, the faculty now has a contextual framework in which to develop a philosophy, conceptual framework, and behavioral objectives that provide the framework, guide, and structure for planning the curriculum and nursing program.

Unit 2

INPUT EVALUATION FOR STRUCTURING DECISIONS; PROCESS EVALUATION FOR IMPLEMENTING DECISIONS

Structuring decisions result in a program's design for student progression in order to meet the curricular objectives. The design is based on the program's philosophy, conceptual framework, and curricular objectives and thereby is unique to each program. Because of the idiosyncratic design or structure of the curriculum, decisions for its implementation distinctive to the program are necessary in order to fulfill its function of providing learning activities.

6

Curricular Design for Learning Activities

The learning activities of the curriculum are organized into a curricular design, a set of courses administered at predetermined times during the year, week, and day (or evening). In developing the design, faculty considers student learning, facilities available for learning, professional and community demands for learning activities, their own qualifications and interests, and the subject matter to be taught, learned, and practiced. The function of the design is the provision for learning experiences, with the goal of the student being the attainment of the objectives as a result of successfully completing the learning activities (courses) within the design.

DEVELOPMENT

Communities

Communities have an influence on the design of a curriculum. One community, as a result of a special health-related task force study of its acute hospital nursing shortage, urged nurse educators to consider offering summer school programs to increase the number of graduates as well as student access to actual experience inside area hospitals (Recruitment of Former Nurses Suggested, The Indianapolis Star, 1979).

Considering the sponsoring institution as a community influence, the university may use as a recruitment tool the fact that the majority of its classes are during the day and on weekdays, thus enabling students to participate in the various cultural and social events offered on or near campus. In such a case, students would come to that institution with this expectation, thus hampering the nursing faculty in its design of the curriculum by necessitating that it be kept within the constraints of days and weekdays.

Clinical Facilities

Clinical facilities used for clinical learning activities are to be considered as the curriculum design is developed. Bevil and Gross (1981) report how a group of faculty used its program objectives as a basis for selecting or evaluating the adequacy of clinical facilities used for student learning. The school's program and level objectives served as the basis for the development of the evaluation instrument because it was "essential to maintain a relationship between learning objectives and clinical facility selection." The instrument was divided into two parts with Part I addressing the clinical facility as a whole: names of contact persons, general restrictions such as maximum number of students per unit and uniform requirements, facilities and resources, location, type of agency, and type of clients. Part II pertained to an individual unit or division within the facility. Each item on the instrument was keyed in the margin with the numbers of the objectives to which it corresponded. One designated faculty member on a biannual basis completed Part I and all clinical faculty members completed Part II every semester.

A survey (Graham and Gleit, 1981) was conducted to obtain a national view of the range of clinical sites used in baccalaureate programs. The sites used by 80 percent or more of the programs were secondary care settings, homes, health departments, outpatient departments, tertiary care settings, schools, and community mental health agencies. Other agencies used, but by a lesser percent of programs, were day-care centers, home health agencies, rehabilitation centers, physician offices, industries, community action programs, Health Maintenance Organizations, jails, summer camps, and long-term facilities.

A common influence on the type of design faculty develops is the availability of clinical facilities. Some facilities that are very desirable may only be available late in the afternoon, evenings or on weekends. This may prompt faculty to provide a weekend or evening program and courses.

If the facilities are available for only short periods (2 to 3 hours), faculty may need to reexamine its whole design (and philosophy) of clinical activities and learning and reduce the activities totally or increase the variety with shorter periods spent in each available area.

Textbooks

An important consideration when developing a course or curriculum design is the availability of the appropriate *level* of textbooks to be used in the curriculum (Ferguson, 1979; Maury-Hess, Cramer, and Bresler, 1979). In one program (Ferguson, 1979), textbooks were analyzed for readability level by the Dale-Chall Readability formula. The national reading skills mean for freshmen entering college is 11th grade and 3 months. The reading skills for the nursing student, according to the analysis of the

TABLE 9. READABILITY LEVELS OF SOME NURSING TEXTS

Text	Title	Author(s)	Edition	Readability Level
Management	The Management of Patient Care	Kron	3rd	11th–12th grade
Dosage and Solution	Dosage and Solution	Blume	2nd	13th–15th grade
Obstetrics	Maternity Nursing	Reader, Mastroianni, Fitzpatrick	13th	13th–15th grade
Psych	Psychiatric Nursing in the Hospital and Community	Burgess, Lazarre	2nd	13th–15th grade
Med–Surg	Medical–Surgical Nursing	Luckmann, Sorensen	1st	13th–15th grade
Pediatrics	Comprehensive Pediatric Nursing	Scipien, et al.	1st	13th–15th grade
Nutrition	Nutrition and Diet Therapy	Williams	2nd	16th, college graduate
Pharmacology	Pharmacology in Nursing	Bergersen	12th	16th, college graduate
Fluid and Electrolyte	Nurses' Handbook of Fluid Balance	Metheny, Snively	2nd	16th, college graduate

(Reprinted from the Journal of Nursing Education, March 1979, Vol. 18, No. 3, p. 7. Published by SLACK Incorporated, Medical Publishers, copyright 1979.)

textbooks, needed to be near the 12th grade level for success to be anticipated (Table 9).

Another program (Maury-Hess et al., 1979) analyzed pediatric and medical–surgical textbooks using the Flesch Formula of readability; the textbooks were at the 13th and 14th grade level for medical–surgical and 10th level for pediatrics. The textbooks analyzed were predominantly used by NLN accredited associate degree programs.

Students

LANGUAGE CODE

Students are a vital consideration in curriculum design development, especially in relation to presentation of content and learning activities. Sayre (1977) discusses the differences of linguistic style and its effect on learning. The student with the restricted linguistic style has a limited command of the language and requires a great deal of attention getting from the instructor before he or she is motivated to be involved in the learning activity. However, the student with the elaborated language code is very symbolic in communication, using complex sentences and verbal relationships. The student with the elaborated language is quite conceptual and abstract and does not require great attention-getting devices to learn. However, the research is revealing that more and more students are bringing a restricted linguistic code with them to postsecondary education, thus requiring higher degrees of attention-getting, creative, innovative teaching strategies from instructors.

MOTIVATION

Along the same line, Gagné (1974) in his theory of instruction suggests that before any learning or apprehending occurs there has to be a motivation phase when the teacher creates an expectancy within the learner. Consideration of the linguistic trend referred to above together with problems of motivation has an effect not only on lecture or seminar material presentation, but on the course and curricular design of the program. Faculty members who organize their curriculum on a wellness–illness continuum may find themselves revising it to an illness–wellness curriculum because of student interest and motivation in wanting to "do" and learn "nursing." Motivation for activity in the sickness–illness arena interferes with students' ability to assimilate wellness concepts at the beginning of a curriculum or nursing program.

STUDENT SUCCESS

Grades. A consideration in design development is grades that are acceptable and unacceptable for student passage and promotion. The university policy is one constraint, but faculty's beliefs are another. A major consideration in the determination of what grades are acceptable is "grade inflation." Bejar (1981) found that grade inflation at the college level is a real phenomenon but it is not a recent one. During the 15 years in Bejar's study, neither the Scholastic Aptitude Test-Verbal (SAT-V) nor the Scholastic Aptitude Test-Math (SAT-M) scores exhibited any increasing tendencies, so it is likely that increases in grade point averages (GPA) at the college level are due to grade inflation, since they have occurred without a concomitant increase in SAT-V and SAT-M scores.

Predictors for Student Progression. When considering student progression in curriculum design development, predictors for success in the curriculum need to be identified. Stronck (1979) found that the first 2 years of student prenursing performance significantly correlated with the last 2 years' GPA of nursing courses, NLN achievement tests, and state boards. A required preadmission essay of the applicant also had a strong positive correlation with future success. An interview correlated negatively while a required reference letter had no correlation.

In another study (Knopke, 1979), significant predictors for success in school were the first semester college GPA and high school percentile rank. Also shown as predictors were the College Qualification Test (CQT) scores of physics, chemistry, and biology and a showing of low order (structure), high dominance (leadership), and high aggression (self-assertiveness) scores on the Edwards Personal Preference Survey (EPPS).

The commitment of the student to the goal of college completion had the strongest positive effect on the decision to remain in the school according to a study by Munro (1981). The educational aspirations of both parents and the student had a greater effect on goal commitment than did academic integration. Academic integration had a much stronger effect on institutional commitment than did social integration.

Eighteen percent of student nurses withdraw between their sophomore and junior year and 19 percent between the junior and senior year as shown by Knopke (1979). Major reasons for leaving were changes in career goals, difficulties with the basic science classes, inability to work with sick people, difficulties in adjusting to school and campus, and failure to maintain the required GPA.

STUDENT–FACULTY RATIO

A more frequent influence on curricular design related to students is the student–faculty ratio. It appears that nursing education can no longer claim "we must be costly to exist." Institutions involved in retrenchment are pressing nursing faculty to show and instigate ways of cost reduction in their programs. Since faculty salaries can be up to 90 percent or more of the budget, faculty reduction is the most significant way of reducing cost and expense. However, the "catch-22" is that the process requires faculty reduction without student reduction and even increased student enrollment.

So, here we have the possibility of 40 students with 2 faculty members where we might previously have had 20 students with 2 faculty members in order to maintain the sacred 1:10 faculty–student ratio. Designs cannot be maintained for 40 students that once supported 20 students. Clinical time for students will need to be evaluated. How much time in the clinical area is needed by the student to meet the objectives? What will the student "do," "develop" while in the clinical area? Infante (1983) has been heard to ask does a student need to bathe a patient every time she or he is in the clinical area to meet the objectives? Infante (1978) also suggests that the faculty–student ratio could easily be 1:16 or even 1:20 if the students were prepared for their clinical assignments; the instructor would be available for guidance but not instruction. She even suggests that the instructor does not need to be in the facility if the students are adequately prepared.

Without a doubt, faculty members will be stretching their innovative, creative minds to develop cost-effective and educationally effective designs to meet the needs and demands of the institution, student, and health care consumer.

STRUCTURE

The structure of the curriculum design is the placement, sequence, and credit allocation of the courses and their prerequisites, the rationale of which is based in the conceptual framework, objectives, and philosophy.

Nonnursing Courses

It has been shown that science courses are a heavy component of the nursing program curriculum. Whether this is based on a conceptual framework or tradition has not been determined. A survey of 53 catalogs of NLN baccalaureate programs in 1978 sought to discover which sciences were most typically represented in current undergraduate nursing curricula and to gather evidence as to whether or not there was systematic inclusion of particular courses (Quiring and Gray, 1979).

On an average during the 4 years of the programs' curricula, there were 21 credits of physiology and biologic sciences, 11 credits of "general education," and 16 credits of "other" which included electives (Quiring and Gray, 1979).

The percentage of baccalaureate programs requiring specified courses were: chemistry 93 percent, microbiology 76 percent, anatomy and physiology 76 percent, biology 43 percent, sociology 77 percent, general education 100 percent, nutrition 64 percent, pharmacology 32 percent,

TABLE 10. EXAMPLE OF COURSES WITHIN APPLIED SCIENCE AND WHOLISTIC NURSING FRAMEWORKS

Nursing Framework:	Nursing is an Applied Science	Nursing is Holistic
Examples of nonnursing courses:	Anatomy & Physiology	Anatomy & Physiology
	Microbiology	Microbiology
	English Composition	English Composition
	Pharmacology	Logic or Philosophy
	Physics	Speech
	Psychology	Human Development
	Abnormal Psychology	English Literature
	Sociology	Cultural Anthropology
	Nutrition	Music, Art Appreciation
	Chemistry	Foreign Language or Culture

statistics 28 percent, and mathematics 25 percent. Twice as much curriculum time was devoted to physical and biologic science as to social science. Upon graduation, nursing students typically had far more science than any science major in a particular field.

Most programs concentrated nursing in the upper division. There was a wide variation in the packaging of the nursing content with the common focus tending to be some aspect of the nursing process. Four sample programs with total and nursing requirement credits were given:

- 120 credits total with 60 credits or 50% nursing
- 180 credits total with 50 credits or 31% nursing
- 188 credits total with 94 credits or 50% nursing
- 190 credits total with 109 credits or 57% nursing

If a conceptual framework is basically a framework of applied physical, social, and psychological sciences, then the nonnursing and nursing courses will support this, with time and credit allocation heavily weighted in those areas. If faculty's conceptualizations of human beings, health, nursing, and environment are very humanistic and holistic in orientation and definition then nonnursing and nursing courses will reflect this, and more emphasis will be placed on liberal arts as well as the physical, social, and psychological sciences (Table 10).

Nursing Courses

Nursing courses come in ranging shapes, sizes, names, and content as one recent study showed (Cantor, Schroeder, and Kurth, 1981). In a survey of new graduates in a hospital setting, in which content in several areas of practice was specifically characterized, only pediatrics as defined

TABLE 11. COURSE TITLES REFLECTING THE CONCEPTUAL FRAMEWORK

Conceptual Framework		Example of Course Titles
Nursing is goal-directed in an illness–wellness continuum	N100	Goals of Nursing
	N120	Restorative Nursing
	N220	Maintenance Nursing
	N320	Promotive Nursing
Persons are bio-psycho-social beings	N200	Medical–Surgical Nursing
	N300	Psychiatric Nursing
	N340	Maternity Nursing
	N400	Pediatric Nursing
		OR
	N101	Holistic Persons
	N200	Nursing the Holistic Person in the Acute Setting
	N300	Nursing the Holistic Person in the Chronic Setting

by the survey had been required for all new graduates in their educational programs; its requirement ranged from 8 to 260 hours of instruction. Maternity experiences ranged from 8 to 260 hours of instruction and general surgery from 4 to 260 hours; some nurses had no experience as students in maternity or general surgery as defined in the survey.

What constitutes the nursing courses is determined by faculty within the framework of the philosophy, conceptual framework, and objectives. The courses will be developed in relation to the sequences of content and learning activities established by faculty. The course titles will reflect the conceptual framework and the sequences as the curriculum progresses through the courses (Table 11).

Each course will reflect the beliefs of the faculty and the identified concepts and conceptual organizers. The level of the course will be reflected in the behaviors of the objectives and the organizing elements placed in the course. Most programs have level objectives that serve as parameters and guides for the establishment of the course objectives. The course overview or outline given to the student will be informative as to behaviors expected, content and concepts to be assimilated, strategies of teaching, and evaluational methods.

Credit Allocation

Obviously, there is no standard method of credit allocation for courses; indeed, the issue is secondary. The most important criterion to follow in curricular development is whether or not the courses are consistent with

N100	Nursing framed in human development	N235	Adolescent
N200	Perinatal	N240	Young adult
N220	Infant	N245	Middle-aged adult
N230	Child	N250	Older adult

Figure 31. Absolute course progression with the framework being human development.

the conceptual framework, objectives, and philosophy of the program. If a faculty has a health continuum-type framework, such as "restoration–maintenance–promotion," the conceptual framework would be the basis for courses, regardless of their titles or basic content arrangement (e.g., medical–surgical nursing versus acute health disruptions) with the organizers in sequence and threaded throughout. The faculty may have small 3- to 4-credit modules of 5 weeks each in rotation or sequence, or large 6- to 10-credit rotating courses. The number of students and faculty help determine credit allocation and the sequence of courses. With a larger number of students and fewer faculty members, inflexible, absolutely progressive course sequence is virtually impossible. To implement such a design, the same faculty would have to teach all the courses in a given year and stay with the same group of students throughout each course, or approximately the same number of students would have to be admitted second semester as first semester in order for there to be students to teach as the first group progresses on to the next course in the sequence. Figure 31 is a good example of inflexible course progression based on a human development framework.

Many schools are dropping the 6- to 12-credit courses and breaking them into smaller units providing increased flexibility and mobility for transfers, registered nurses (RNs), working students, and repeaters and relieving students from being saddled with a large amount of credit for one course.

So, the trend for credit allocation is courses with 2, 3 or 4 credits each (usually including clinical within that credit allocation) and limited constraints on the sequence in which the courses are taken.

Special Programs

Curriculum designs are often punctuated with special courses and special programs such as remedial courses and cultural socialization programs. One such program was an affirmative action program that focused upon promoting the success of minority students in a baccalaureate nursing program (Story, 1978). Before the students' freshman year, they had a

10-week noncredit summer program which included reading, writing, and studying skills, skills in test taking, review of math skills, relaxation therapy, and assertiveness training. While freshmen during the first quarter, the students met with counselors weekly for self-assessment and referral and for tutorial academic assistance. During the second quarter, they continued to meet weekly for self-assessment with the counselor and had bi-monthly group sessions with all other prenursing students in the special program.

During the third quarter, the self-assessment was individual with continued group sessions and academic counseling. At this time the minority student was assigned a "big sister" in the nursing program for peer support.

The summer before the sophomore year a 10-week noncredit session dealt with the following topics: introduction to nursing, the nursing process, learning how to learn from a module, and an introduction to psychomotor nursing skills. The special sophomore year program provided a review of anatomy and physiology, an introductory course in the body systems, individual conferences, and bi-monthly group process meetings with academic tutoring as needed.

After the senior year, there was a 10-week preparation for state boards.

This was a planned, systematic curriculum design for minority students superimposed upon the nursing program's curriculum design. Such programs can be this systematic or more informal. Most have an effect, predictably positive, upon the student as she or he progresses in the program (Kulik, Kulik, and Shwalb, 1983).

Alternate Designs: For the First Professional Degree

The three alternate designs reviewed here will be the modified programs that enable registered nurses to acquire a baccalaureate degree in nursing, the external degree program, and the programs of postbaccalaureate masters and doctorates as the first professional degree.

REGISTERED NURSE-BACHELOR OF SCIENCE IN NURSING DEGREE (RN-BSN)

The ANA has entreated nursing educators to provide flexible opportunities for nurses (RNs) seeking academic degrees in nursing (American Nurses Association, 1978; Resolution 53, 1980). The NLN states that "educational institutions are responsible for setting policies on admissions, graduation, and transfers of credits" for those wishing educational mobility. "In a plan for educational mobility, opportunity should be provided for students to validate previously acquired education and clinical competencies to facilitate advanced placement" (National League for Nursing, 1982). The demand of RN students seeking BSN degrees is substantial. The American Association of Colleges of Nursing (AACN) found an increase in enrollment of part-time nursing students, particularly registered nurses seeking baccalaureate degrees in nursing, when there was overall a 5 percent decline in the number of full-time (generic) students enrolled in 4-year nursing programs.

RN Student in the Generic Program. One method of RN-BSN education is the incorporation of the RN into a generic program. Parlocha and Hiraki (1982) warn that in the generic program that admits RN students "faculty must be aware of two basic assumptions before implementing any teaching strategy. First, RN students are different from generic students" usually requiring adult education principles and "second, RN students require more faculty time than generic students. . . . When the RN attempts to make the transition back to the role of student in the university setting, there is an effect called academic shock" (Parlocha and Hiraki, 1982, p. 23). As faculty members become aware of the academic shock phenomenon and the different learning styles of the RN, adult learning strategies become incorporated into the RN-BSN track within the generic program.

When planning a program for the RN student in the generic program, a formal orientation for incoming RN students is usually provided. The orientation is in the form of a workshop or course designed for RNs which addresses the conceptual framework, concepts, and subconcepts of the subject matter and problem-solving strategies expected to be used by the RN throughout the program. The content of this course determined by the faculty to be necessary for entry into the nursing courses becomes the basis for the entire curriculum and remains present throughout the program (Borgman and Ostrow, 1981; Parlocha and Hiraki, 1982; Roy, 1979). This introductory course is similar in content to the introductory course for the generic student except for the omission of skill development.

Advanced placement examination over some or all of the courses may be an option the faculty provides for the RN student at the completion of the introductory course. This may be accomplished by case studies, teacher-made or standardized tests or a combination thereof. In general, since courses require of students both content and laboratory activities to meet the course objectives, it is logical that placement testing of the RN would also require content and laboratory evaluation (Dean and Edwards, 1982; Gross and Bevil, 1981). Placement testing determines whether or not the RNs can apply the newly learned concepts, conceptual framework, and problem-solving skills to familiar, previously learned content. It is the faculty's decision to determine, within the guidelines of its institution, how many courses the RN may pass through special examination. Usually the "basic" courses are available for testing out. Actual enrollment in courses such as "advanced nursing," "community health," and "management" are required for the RN in order to complete the requirements necessary to achieve the objectives of the program for graduation.

The RN enrolled in the generic program attains the same objectives of the same courses as the generic student. The requirements may be attained by way of testing-out, a special track for RNs that incorporates androgogic principles or by way of enrollment in the courses with the generic student. Upon graduation, the RN and the generic student have a common conceptual framework and philosophy.

RN Student in the RN-BSN Program. The other major RN-BSN program is the upper division program only for RNs. In this type of program, the RN student's records are usually reviewed by faculty to determine if any of the academic program can be transferred for the BSN, although much of the responsibility for the transferability of credits is that of the registrar. After the records have been reviewed, faculty administers standardized content and performance tests to determine acceptance and an entry level into the program. Once entry behaviors have been evaluated and attained by the RN, the curriculum is entered. Upon completion of the curriculum, the student is granted the BSN, having met the general education and nursing curricular requirements of the institution and of the professional accrediting body.

The curricula of the RN-BSN programs are as varied as the day is long. Most generally the basic courses of adult, pediatric, psychiatric, and maternity nursing are not offered. Programs traditionally offer courses in leadership, management, and community health. Some programs include practitioner and assessment skills as a major component. Regardless of the specifics of the curriculum, the RN graduates, as all graduates of BSN programs, a generalist and a professional practitioner.

Socialization of the RN. RNs in a BSN program, whether generic or nontraditional, experience culture shock in the returning-to-school syndrome (Shane, 1980; Woolley, 1978). There is at first a honeymoon phase which is pleasant but terminates during the time the RN is enrolled in the first class that contains substantial nursing content and practice. The RN experiences conflict, with a growing sense of becoming different. There is hostility with a strong rejection of the new culture of the baccalaureate program. There are two dead-end resolutions to the conflict: one is a false acceptance with bottled-up emotion and the other is a chronic hostility. The promoted and desired end of schooling is biculturalism, a resocialization and an alignment with the profession as a professional nurse; the RN becomes a manager, health promoter and supervisor, health screener, teacher and counselor, as well as a care-giver (Kramer, 1981).

Academic Mobility. An unsettled issue concerning the RN-BSN programs is the issue of mobility and whether indeed nursing education should provide it. Montag (Ingles and Montag, 1971) comments about the concept of ladder, "upward" mobility, remarking that the profession should dignify kinds or types of nursing practice that it has, rather than see them as levels or rungs on a ladder to some place else. Montag goes on to say that if "professional curriculums in nursing concentrate the major offerings at the upper division level, and if these offerings are in fact upper divisional and professional in content and method, few would be likely to challenge successfully. If any number are successful, then one would be forced to question the character of both programs" (Ingles and Montag, 1971, p. 729).

As long as there is controversy over the level of entry into practice, ladder upward mobility will be present out of sheer pressure from the student wanting and perhaps feeling pressure to attain the advanced degree. There are limited ways educators can prevent a person from seeking further education regardless of whether each level of education is respected or not. The trend appears to be with the request of the professional organizations to provide advanced study mobility to the RN within her own professional discipline. It is the responsibility of the faculties of nursing not to become mere credentialing agencies but to educate for a high professionalism. Nurses educated in professional nursing can do nothing less than fortify and edify the health care system.

EXTERNAL DEGREE

The external degree programs focus on the concept of providing credit on the basis of what one knows, not on how one has achieved it (Sims, 1978). An external degree is awarded on the basis of the program of study not centered on the traditional patterns of residential or university study.

A well-known external degree program in nursing is the one offered by the University of the State of New York: the New York Regents External Degree Program offering the Bachelor of Science in Nursing and the Associate Degree in Nursing (College Proficiency Examinations Regents External Degree, 1978). "The Regents External Degree, as an assessment program, offers no instruction or supervised clinical experience" (College Proficiency Examinations Regents External Degree, 1978, p. 11).

In order to earn an associate of science in nursing degree, the student must fulfill the requirements in two components: general education and nursing. The general education component requires 30 semester hours, all in liberal arts and sciences. It can be met by a "combination of college courses, proficiency examinations, military education courses, noncollegiate sponsored courses or special assessment" (College Proficiency Examinations Regents External Degree, 1978, p. 12). The nursing component is divided into four areas: nursing health care, commonalities in nursing care, differences in nursing care, and occupational strategy. Seven objective examinations covering these four areas are required. The student must also pass a clinical performance examination in a hospital setting. The 2-1/2 day examination tests abilities in planning, implementing, and evaluating nursing care for several different patients.

The BSN requires 72 hours in general education consisting of humanities, social studies, natural science, mathematics, and unrestricted electives. The nursing component is divided into 6 examinations: health restoration, health supports, professional strategies, clinical performance, health assessment performance, and professional performance.

Most state boards of nursing and university schools of nursing now accept the external degree as a legitimate degree. The degrees from the New York Regents are accredited by the National League for Nursing. The graduate has attained the objectives of the ASN or BSN degree, with the difference between external degree and a residential degree being the method of attainment, not the outcome.

POSTBACCALAUREATE PROFESSIONAL DEGREE

Master's Degree. The hospital diploma, the associate of science, and bachelor of science degrees in nursing have been the most popular initial preparation (generic) for the nurse. Now available for the first professional degree are the master of nursing and the nursing doctorate for initial preparation and entry into the nursing profession. Slavinsky and Diers (1982) describe the master's level postbaccalaureate professional degree for the nonnurses at Yale University as a 3-year curriculum which not only prepares nurses, but nurses who can function in advanced practice specialty roles as nurse midwife, nurse practitioner or clinical nurse specialist. The Yale degree gives students the option to progress through both basic and advanced nursing without a break or interim degree by awarding the MSN as the first professional degree at the master's level. Some programs offer an MN which does not include the extra credits toward a specialty.

Nursing Doctorate Degree. The Doctor of Nursing Degree (ND) at Frances Payne Bolton School of Nursing at Case Western Reserve University provides a broad and sound knowledge base for clinical nursing practice; provides for equitable preparation for the three practice settings of primary, long-term, and acute care; emphasizes utilization of research findings through scientific inquiry as a contribution to nursing knowledge; and provides opportunity for learning collaborative and interdependent practice with other health professionals (The New Dimension: The Doctor of Nursing Degree). "The graduate will emerge fully prepared to utilize research findings as a basis for practicing, to identify problems for investigation and to participate in research endeavors" (The New Dimension: The Doctor of Nursing Degree, p. 8). These objectives are accomplished and the competence of the graduate increased during a period of concentrated study and increasingly independent practice during the last year of the program.

Whether the ND or MN/MSN will ever be the generally accepted preparation for the first level of entry into practice remains to be seen. There are more programs offering the master's degree as the first level of preparation than there were 10 years ago. However, since we still have three levels of programs lower than the master's offering preparation for entry into practice, it may be some time until we recognize the graduate degrees as initial preparation for entry into practice.

FUNCTION

The function of the curriculum design is the provision of learning activities which enable students to meet the objectives of the program. Using again Joyce and Weil's (1980) categories of learning, we may discuss the four major types of learning activities and teaching strategies used in the curriculum.

Conditioning

The teaching strategy used for the outcome of conditioning is associational or quantitative accumulation. This teaching entails learning in sequences or small stages with frequent reinforcement. Conditional learning

Programmed instruction	Assertiveness training
Relaxation techniques	Skill practice for proficiency
Role modeling	Stress reduction exercises
Desensitization for anxiety	Memorizing

Figure 32. Learning activities for conditioning.

Inquiry training	Essays
Journals	Problem-solving sessions
Concept analysis	Term papers
Peer teaching	Patient care plans
Small group discussion	Patient care
Postconferences	Teacher–student dyad
Research project	Class presentations

Figure 33. Learning activities for information processing.

can occur through programmed instruction, computer-assisted instruction, role modeling, lecturing, and reading. Examples of conditioned learning are cardiopulmonary resuscitation (CPR) training or any skill training, and any memorizing of content for mere recall or repetition. Before evaluation of conditioned behavior, the student requires conditioning learning opportunities: practice and memorization (Fig. 32).

Information Processing

Teaching strategies for information processing include conceptual rather than factual development of content, such as essays, journals, term papers, peer teaching, problem-solving inquiry sessions, and small group discussions. A specific example of information-processing learning activity is the thinking that occurs when the student is performing client care and relevant discussion with faculty and peers follows. Little use of memorization is required other than that which is used as a basis for the analysis, synthesis, and evaluation involved in client care (Fig. 33).

Games		Simulations
Group dynamic sessions		Roleplaying
Group projects:	Health fairs	
	Health screening	
	Research/investigation	

Figure 34. Learning activities for social interaction.

Awareness training	Creativity exercises
Poem, prose construction	Values clarification
Ethical dilemma sessions	Encounter groups
Journals	Role playing
Free expression exercises	Growth games

Figure 35. Learning activities for personal awareness.

Social Interaction

Teaching strategies for social interaction involve group dynamic sessions, games, simulations, and group projects. Specific examples include any group project done by the students. Health fairs and health screening developed and implemented by students are good examples of learning experiences for the purpose of meeting social interaction objectives (Fig. 34).

Personal Awareness

Teaching strategies of personal awareness include personal development workshops, values clarification sessions, ethical dilemma decisions, role playing, and construction of poems, prose, and journals. Examples of personal awareness behaviors are self-evaluation and self-disclosure.

After the curriculum is developed, the student progresses through a preplanned sequence or rotation of learning activities in order to reach and attain the objectives of the program. The curriculum design provides the structures for student progression and its function is the provision of learning activities for that progression (Fig. 35).

REFERENCES

American Nurses Association. *Statement on flexible patterns of nursing education.* American Nurses Association Publication NE-3, 1978.

Bejar, I. I., & Blew, E. O. Grade inflation and the validity of the Scholastic Aptitude Test. *Amer Educ Research J,* 1981, 18, 143–156.

Bevil, C. W., & Gross, L. D. Assessing the adequacy of clinical learning settings. *Nurs Outlook,* 1981, 29, 658–661.

Borgman, M. F., & Ostrow, C. L. An advanced placement program for registered nurses. *J Nurs Educ,* 1981, 20, 2–6.

Cantor, M. M., Schroeder, D. M., & Kurth, S. W. The experienced nurse and the new graduate: Do their learning needs differ? *Nurse Educator,* 1981, 6, 248–250.

College Proficiency Examinations Regents External Degree, New York: The University of the State of New York, 1978.

Dean, P. R., & Edwards, T. A. A multidimensional approach to evaluation. *J Nurs Educ,* 1982, 21, 18–23.

Ferguson, C. K. Reading skills versus success in nursing school. *J Nurs Educ,* 1979, 18, 6–12.

Gagné, R. M. *Essentials of Learning for Instruction.* Hinsdale, Illinois: Dryden Press, 1974.

Graham, B. A., & Gleit, C. J. Clinical sites used in baccalaureate programs. *Nurs Outlook,* 1981, 29, 291–294.

Gross. L., & Bevil, C. The use of testing to modify curricula for RNs. *Nurs Outlook,* 1981, 29, 541–545.

Infante, M. S. *Creative clinical teaching.* Paper presented at the Northwest Indiana Nursing Education Program's Consortium, October, 1983.

Infante, M. S. Meeting program objectives in the clinical laboratory. In NLN Publication, *Utilization of the Clinical Laboratory in Baccalaureate Nursing Programs.* New York: National League for Nursing Publication 15-1726, 1978.

Ingles, T., & Montag, M. Debate: Ladder concept in nursing education. *Nurs Outlook,* 1971, 19, 726–730.

Joyce, B., & Weil, M. *Models of Teaching* (2nd ed.). Englewood Cliffs, N.J.: Prentice-Hall, 1980.

Knopke, H. J. Predicting student attrition in a baccalaureate curriculum. *Nurs Research,* 1979, 28, 224–227.

Kramer, M. Philosophical foundations of baccalaureate nursing education. *Nurs Outlook,* 1981, 29, 224–228.

Kulik, C. C., Kulik, J. A., & Shwalb, B. J. College programs for high-risk and disadvantaged students. A Meta-analysis of findings. *Rev Educ Research,* 1983, 53, 397–414.

Maury-Hess, S., Crancer, J., & Bresler, M. Textbook selection for Associate Degree nursing programs (an evaluative study). *J Nurs Educ,* 1979, 18, 11–16.

Munro, B. H. Dropouts from higher education: Path analysis of a national sample. *Am Educ Research J,* 1981, 18, 133–141.

National League for Nursing. *Position Statement on Educational Mobility.* New York: National League for Nursing Publication 11-1892, 1982.

Nursing enrollment drops 5 percent in 2 years. *Chron Higher Educ,* 1982, 24, p. 10.

Parlocha, P., & Hiraki, A. Strategies for faculty: Teaching the RN student in a BSN program. *J Nurs Educ,* 1982, 21, 22–25.

Quiring, J. D., & Gray, G. T. Is baccalaureate education based on a patchwork curriculum? *Nurs Outlook,* 1979, 27, 708–713.

Recruitment of former nurses suggested. *The Indianapolis Star,* December 1979, p. 71.

Resolution 53: 1980 American Nurses Association Convention. *Am Nurse,* July–August 1980, p. 13.

Roy, A. L. The placement process. *Nurse Educator,* 1979, 4, 14–18.

Sayre, J. The role of linguistic style in student learning difficulties. *J Nurs Educ,* 1977, 16, 16–23.

Shane, D. L. The returning-to-school syndrome. In S. K. Mirin (Ed.), *Teaching Tomorrow's Nurse: A Nurse Educator Reader.* Wakefield, Massachusetts: Nursing Resources, 1980.

Sims, L. A. Perspective: The external degree as a viable education model in nursing. *J Nurs Educ,* 1978, 17, 23–27.

Slavinsky, A. T., & Diers, D. Nursing education for college graduates. *Nurs Outlook,* 1982, 30, 292–297.

Story, B. W. The I AM model for retention of minority nursing students. *Nurse Educator,* 1978, 3, 16–20.

Stronck, D. Predicting performance from college admission criteria. *Nurs Outlook,* 1979, 27, 604–607.

The New Dimension: The Doctor of Nursing Degree. Cleveland: Frances Payne Bolton School of Nursing, Case Western Reserve University.

Woolley, A. S. From RN to BSN: Faculty perceptions. *Nurs Outlook,* 1978, 26, 103–108.

7

Conclusion of Unit 2

AN EXAMPLE OF INPUT EVALUATION FOR STRUCTURING DECISIONS

Questions Asked for Data Gathering	*Sources of Data*
What are the constraints of the sponsoring institution as to day, evening, weekend classes?	1. University catalog 2. University recruitment pamphlets
How are the courses to be sequenced?	1. Conceptual framework of nursing program
Where lies student interest in what course comes first?	1. Survey of students in beginning of program of what they are eager to learn and have 2. Survey of students in the program as to what they wished the sequence of the courses were 3. Survey of graduates as to recommendations for course sequencing
How many credits should be assigned to nursing courses?	1. University policy 2. Faculty survey for opinion and philosophy 3. Literature review for relative comparisons and data 4. Objectives of courses 5. University schedule's flexibility to credits desired

Do courses include a clinical component or is one course clinical and an accompanying course content?	1. Survey of faculty opinion 2. Literature review 3. University policy
Once the nursing courses are established, are there clinical facilities to provide the learning activities required to meet the objectives of the courses?	1. Survey of clinical facilities in town, city and out of town, city, county for a. availability b. when available c. whether they meet criteria for state board 2. Use of criteria established by Bevil and Gross (1981) 3. Clinical facilities wanted by faculty 4. State Board of Health facility assessments of counties
What textbooks should be used for the courses?	1. Review of literature (book reviews in literature) 2. Review of Maury-Hess et al. (1979) and Ferguson (1979) 3. Review of table of contents of possible texts
What will be the student–faculty ratio?	1. Survey of faculty's beliefs about learning related to student–faculty ratio 2. Workshop on teaching strategies for decided-upon ratio 3. Facilities' parameters on number of students and time students can be there
How prepared is faculty for the students with low interest, low motivation, and restricted language style?	1. Educational vitae of faculty members to determine if any have had teaching strategies courses 2. Workshop on teaching strategies

What is faculty's belief about passing and satisfactory grades, i.e., is C− the lowest passing grade for nursing and nonnursing required courses? C? D?	1. Survey of faculty 2. Small group discussion of faculty 3. University policy 4. Literature review of what other programs do
How can faculty predict student's success in program?	1. High school GPA 2. High school rank 3. College GPA 4. EPPS 5. Student's commitment to goal of college completion
What nonnursing required courses should students take?	1. University requirements in university catalog 2. Conceptual framework as basis for nonnursing required courses 3. Survey of faculty about courses based on the conceptual framework 4. Pooling faculty suggestions and resubmitting 5. Committee finalizes list for faculty approval 6. University catalog to see if suggested nonnursing courses are offered
How can the nursing program meet needs of the learner in relation to its design?	1. Policy of university about summer school, weekend sessions 2. Willingness of faculty to teach evenings, weekends, summers
What is available for the student with ability, but without study skills or substantial academic background?	1. University counseling center 2. Study skill laboratory availability 3. Public/community study skill laboratories 4. Survey of faculty and students interested in providing tutoring 5. Tutoring availability in university (e.g., Mortar Board)
What to do about the RN student?	1. Survey of faculty's beliefs about accepting RNs into program

	2. Feasibility study of community if RNs are interested in coming to program for degree 3. Literature review of what to do with and about RNs 4. Workshops of what to do with and about RNs. (University of Texas, San Antonio, e.g., has had workshops in 1983 and 1984.)
How should faculty be distributed between generic and RN?	1. Ask faculty 2. Review of literature 3. Financial resource availability for full-time RN advisor/coordinaιor

STRUCTURING DECISIONS

The data gathered for input evaluation provide enough information for structuring the curriculum in form of a design. The curriculum is now ready for implementation with student progression.

AN EXAMPLE OF PROCESS EVALUATION FOR IMPLEMENTING DECISIONS

Questions Asked for Data Gathering	*Sources of Data*
What is the attrition/retention rate of students?	1. Statistics after each course or year of a. number of students withdrawn, dismissed, dropped-out b. reasons for above
How do nursing students' grades compare to nonnursing students' grades?	1. From registrar, statistics of mean grades for nonnursing and nursing courses, mean grades of colleges, departments
What is the morale of faculty and students?	1. Morale, motivation studies 2. Statistics on number of students and faculty formally complaining about program, and frequency

Are the students progressing through program smoothly? Are they meeting course objectives?	1. Course-repeat rate by students 2. Mean grades of courses 3. Mean grades on unit exams 4. Course evaluation of students 5. Observation to determine if teaching strategies coincide with objectives 6. Faculty evaluation of own course
Can transfer students come into program of nursing? Is an accelerated track possible?	1. Transferable credits determined by registrar 2. Faculty survey on acceptance of accelerated track and potential unevenness and limited predictability of numbers of students in each course
Are the organizing elements evident in courses?	1. Course outlines 2. Grid of elements with course outline and objectives
How are the clinical facilities reacting to the number of students and the time of their presence?	1. Outreach meetings every semester with clinical faculty and clinical facility personnel for data gathering purposes and information giving
Do courses lead to terminal objectives?	1. Grid of terminal objectives with course and level objectives
How does faculty feel and what does it think about the implementation of the program?	1. Faculty–director–curriculum chairperson conference (dyad or triad) 2. Faculty team meetings 3. Faculty small group discussion 4. Faculty meeting
What do students think and feel about the program?	1. Student–director and/or student–advisee dyad 2. Student–faculty small group discussion 3. Student survey with list of objectives, courses, conceptual framework, assignments and other data to which to react

	4. Class presidents gather information in class meetings
Are textbooks satisfactory?	1. Part of course evaluation by students 2. Faculty assessment during and at conclusion of course
Are clinical facilities adequate for student learning?	1. Use of tool (Bevil and Gross, 1981) 2. Outreach meetings
What is the best faculty–student ratio?	1. Survey of faculty 2. Share survey results in small group discussions 3. Compare with literature about other programs and research 4. Elicit reaction from clinical facility personnel in outreach meetings
Does the faculty still think the nonnursing required courses should be what they are?	1. Concept analysis of nonnursing required courses with program conceptual framework and objectives 2 Analysis of prerequisites to nursing courses 3. Analysis of courses needed to meet terminal objectives
Should the progression of courses still be as faculty originally proposed?	1. Readiness of students by pretests in courses 2. Prerequisites of each course 3. Reevaluation of conceptual elements sequencing
Is the number of credits appropriate for each course? Should nursing content and clinical be separate credit courses?	1. Objectives of courses versus credit allocation 2. Number of hours of clinical versus credit allocation

IMPLEMENTING DECISIONS

Process evaluation provides data about the implementation of the program; from these data faculty becomes aware of the weaknesses and strengths of the curriculum.

Unit 3

PRODUCT EVALUATION FOR RECYCLING DECISIONS

Recycling decisions deals with whether or not to maintain or revise the curriculum. All program aspects related to the curriculum are measured and evaluated in a systematic manner. Once the worth of the curriculum and its parts is determined and the need for change has been established, recycling occurs by way of incremental, metamorphic or neomobilistic processes.

8

Evaluation

The last phase of curriculum development is product evaluation, which not only serves its own valid purposes but initiates context evaluation and therefore the evaluation of the entire educational process (Clark et al., 1983).

DEVELOPMENT

Product evaluation does not occur just when the student graduates but is a continuous process beginning with data covering the entering student and extending beyond the time of graduation. Important pieces of data in product evaluation are the prediction indicators for graduation, admission requirements, and related information: demography of students, GPA of high school, prenursing and nonnursing courses, preadmission scores and admission policy which may be open, closed or selected. These data describe the entering student (McMorrow, 1978; Yess, 1980). At the other end, data for product evaluation include state board examination scores, program evaluation by students immediately upon graduation and years afterward, studies of the effects of liberal studies, attitude development and socialization, and studies of recruitment effectiveness (recruitment–admission–retention and graduation comparisons) (Clayton and Triplett, 1981; Fields, 1979; Mays, 1979; Melcolm et al., 1981; Packard et al., 1979; Stroller, 1978).

According to Stake, continuous and constant product evaluation involves examining the countenance of the curriculum design and all its components. Evaluation can be related to Popham and Tyler's attainment of objectives; Scriven's effectiveness—primary, secondary, and tertiary; Stake's program congruency and contingency; and Stuffelbeam's planning, structuring, implementing, and recycling decisions (Worthen and Sanders, 1973; House, 1978).

STRUCTURE

The structure of evaluation is a grid or form incorporating but not necessarily delineating the philosophy, conceptual framework, and objectives designating the terms of measurement and data to be collected to be used for evaluation. The evaluation grid suggests a set of questionnaires, surveys, and other related measurement tools relating to administration, courses, faculty, students, and facilities, and the time frame in which each should be measured and evaluated. The data from the measurement tools then lead to the initiation of the whole process of judgment, evaluation, and decision making determining curriculum maintenance—homeostasis, or revision—incremental (improvement changes), neomobilistic (quick changes), and metamorphic (complete changes) (Stuffelbeam, in Worthen and Sanders, 1973).

Models of Evaluation

CIPP MODEL

The evaluation grid or form can be structured after one of several models (Worthen and Sanders, 1973). One model frequently used is Stuffelbeam's CIPP evaluation model (Clark et al., 1983; National League for Nursing, 1978; Steele, 1978; Worthen and Sanders, 1978). The CIPP model is a four-step model of program evaluation developed for the purpose of obtaining useful information for making decisions. It involves context evaluation for planning decisions, input evaluation for structuring decisions, process evaluation for implementing decisions, and product evaluation for recycling decisions. Product evaluation leads to the reinitiation of context evaluation.

Within each step or stage of the CIPP model, the data are delineated, obtained, and reported for decisions to be made. This curriculum text has used the CIPP model for curriculum development. At each step it has been determined what data should be collected, how data should be obtained, and to whom and how data are to be reported for decisions to be made. Figure 36 illustrates in a capsule the use of the CIPP model for program evaluation. It is an adaptation of the CIPP model in Worthen and Sanders (1973).

COUNTENANCE MODEL

Stake's model of program evaluation is a countenance model in which the emphasis is on the collection of descriptive and judgmental data (Ediger et al., 1983; Marriner et al., 1980; Worthen and Sanders, 1973). Data can be collected through direct observation, interviews, questionnaires, check lists, records, tests, as well as from other legitimate sources.

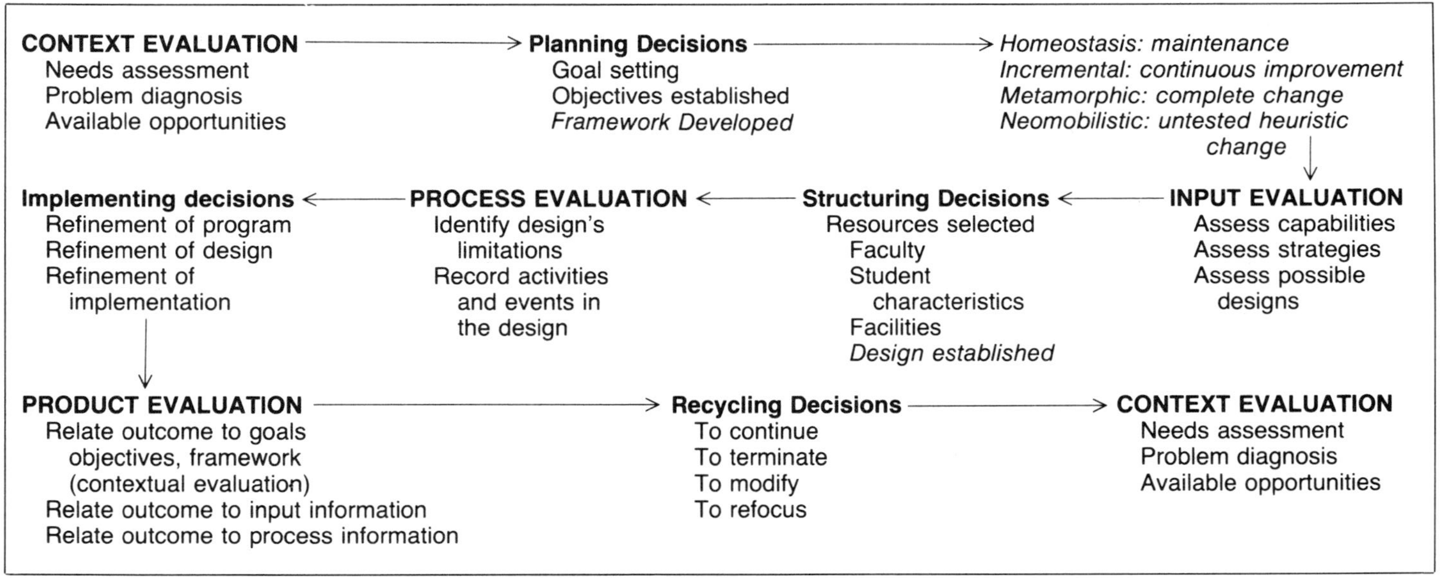

CONTEXT EVALUATION →
Needs assessment
Problem diagnosis
Available opportunities

Planning Decisions →
Goal setting
Objectives established
Framework Developed

Homeostasis: maintenance
Incremental: continuous improvement
Metamorphic: complete change
Neomobilistic: untested heuristic change ↓

INPUT EVALUATION →
Assess capabilities
Assess strategies
Assess possible designs

Structuring Decisions →
Resources selected
Faculty
Student characteristics
Facilities
Design established

PROCESS EVALUATION →
Identify design's limitations
Record activities and events in the design

Implementing decisions ↓
Refinement of program
Refinement of design
Refinement of implementation

PRODUCT EVALUATION →
Relate outcome to goals objectives, framework (contextual evaluation)
Relate outcome to input information
Relate outcome to process information

Recycling Decisions →
To continue
To terminate
To modify
To refocus

CONTEXT EVALUATION
Needs assessment
Problem diagnosis
Available opportunities

Figure 36. CIPP model of program evaluation.

	INTENTS		OBSERVATION	STANDARDS		JUDGMENTS
				Absolute	*Relative*	
Antecedents						
Logical contingency	Desired student characteristics Desired level of students Faculty interest, expertise	Empirical contingency	Data collected through EPPS Questionnaires Demographics Faculty vita	National norms of 75 percentile SAT-V, SAT-M NLN criteria for faculty EPPS results reported in literature	Standards of another program	Descriptive matrix is compared to standards of judgment matrix and judgments are made related to the antecedents, transactions and outcomes of the nursing program.
	----congruence----					
Transactions						
	Curriculum design Student–teacher interactions Student progression		Data collected through Faculty, course, student evaluations Unit, course examinations	Nursing theorist model of nursing NLN criteria related to curriculum	Standards of another program	

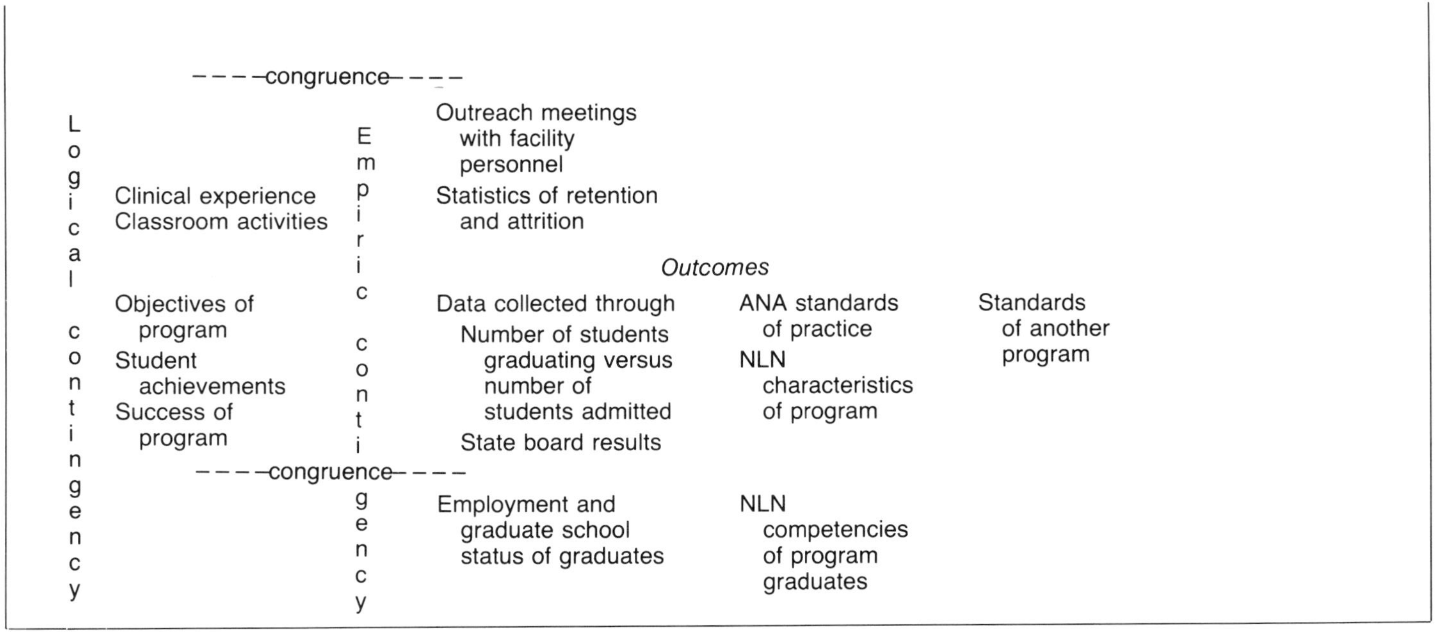

---- congruence ----

Logical contingency

Empirical contingency

Clinical experience
Classroom activities

Outreach meetings with facility personnel
Statistics of retention and attrition

Outcomes

Objectives of program
Student achievements
Success of program

Data collected through
Number of students graduating versus number of students admitted
State board results

ANA standards of practice
NLN characteristics of program

Standards of another program

---- congruence ----

Employment and graduate school status of graduates

NLN competencies of program graduates

Figure 37. Countenance model for program evaluation.

The data are distributed among three areas: antecedents or objectives, transactions or processes, and outcomes or product; two matrices are used for the evaluation process.

The descriptive matrix includes two columns—the intents of the faculty and observations of what actually happened. The contingency relationship of the intended antecedents, transactions, and product is determined by logical reasoning; the contingency relationship between the observed antecedents, transactions, and product is determined by empiric evidence. The congruency between the intents and the observations is determined by measuring what occurred to what was intended.

The judgment matrix involves comparing the descriptive matrix to a standard. Processing the judgment matrix data involves comparing the observed antecedents, transactions, and outcomes with standardized criteria (National League for Nursing, 1982, 1983) or with relative criteria (a similar program or programs). Figure 37 illustrates the use of Stake's countenance model for program evaluation.

BEHAVIORAL OBJECTIVE MODEL

A very common model of evaluation, but one found not to provide a complete program evaluation, is the behavioral objective model proposed by Tyler, Popham, and Hammond (National League for Nursing, 1978; Worthen and Sanders, 1973). The method of the behavioral objectives model is to judge the failure or success of a program on its graduates meeting the curriculum's behavioral objectives. Obviously, this is limited in scope and denies evaluation from input and process data, not to mention the evaluation of the behavioral objectives themselves (context evaluation). The behavioral objectives model is manageable and worthwhile, though, when evaluation of whether the program (or course, unit, lesson) objectives have been attained by the students is of primary and immediate concern (Fig. 38).

GOAL-FREE MODEL

Another model for evaluation, but more in an abstract, philosophic sense than a directive sense, is the goal-free model of Scriven (National League for Nursing, 1978; Worthen and Sanders, 1973). This model studies the effectiveness of the program from the standpoint of both expected and unexpected and formative and summative effects. Goals or objectives are considered, but only in relation to the effects of the program. The effects are three-tiered and interrelated: primary effects are those most closely related to what is being evaluated—students, curriculum, faculty, graduates; secondary effects are affected by the primary effects—the con-

Program objectives:	Data ⟶ measured to objectives
Level objectives:	Data ⟶ measured to objectives
Course objectives:	Data ⟶ measured to objectives
Unit objectives:	Data ⟶ measured to objectives
Class objectives:	Data ⟶ measured to objectives
Clinical day (week) objectives:	Data ⟶ measured to objectives

Data collected to determine if objectives have been attained.
Judgment made.

Figure 38. Evaluation by objectives.

sumer (service, graduate programs), community; the tertiary effects are affected by the secondary effects—the profession, health care. An expert (usually external to the program) in evaluation needs to be involved in determining what effects are to be studied and what data need to be collected for examination (Fig. 39).

Whatever the model or combination of models chosen and used, it provides a systematic and conceptualized measurement process in its structure. An evaluation model provides a complete, ongoing evaluation of a program based on its philosophy, conceptual framework and objectives.

Table 12 summarizes each of the models of evaluation presented.

FUNCTION

The function of evaluation is to determine the worth of the curriculum as well as the program in general. Evaluation applies to the administrative structure and governance, resources, policies, faculty, and curriculum, all in the light of the philosophy, conceptual framework, and objectives (National League of Nursing, 1983).

Since evaluations function to determine worth, the whole question of the significance, reliability, and validity of tests and measurements surfaces. "Fair" evaluation of administration, faculty, students, a unit, course or curriculum involves subjective judgment based on objective data. When the philosophy, conceptual framework, and objectives are used as the context and standard of evaluation, the measurement and

	Formative	Summative
Primary effects of program	Level, course, unit objectives reached by students (cognitive, affective, motor)	Terminal objectives reached by graduates (cognitive, affective, motor)
	Course, instructor evaluations	Success in employment and/or graduate school of graduates
	Are the organizing elements being assimilated and internalized?	Program evaluation by students, consumer, accrediting body
		Did integration of conceptual framework occur?
Secondary effects of program	What have instructors done resulting from student, peer, administration evaluations?	How has the program changed as a result of graduates' evaluation?
	How are courses different as a result of student evaluations?	Are the terminal objectives still satisfactory?
	Should courses, organizing elements still be sequenced as originally planned?	
Tertiary effects of program	How are clinical facilities affected by students' and faculty's presence?	Have graduates effected change in their place of employment?
	What changes have occurred in the facilities as a result of the nursing program's influence?	Are the faculty or graduates getting requests for inservice from employers of graduates?
	Have other departments/colleges within the university developed policies, protocols, patterning after the college of nursing?	

Figure 39. Goal-free evaluation model.

evaluation tend to be more consistent and defensible than if no framework were used. Flaskerud (1983) discovered that when the conceptual framework and objectives served as a base for clinical evaluation tools the clinical evaluation tools developed for all courses turned out to be the same conceptually. The same could be true for all evaluation tools within the curriculum and nursing program (unit and course examinations, care plans, process recordings, and journals) if the philosophy, objectives, and conceptual framework were the basis for their development. Stuffelbeam suggests that the function of product evaluation is to make decisions as to whether to "continue, terminate, modify or refocus a program" and Provus suggests that the function is to "determine whether to improve, maintain, or terminate a program" (Worthen and Sanders, 1973, p. 210). Therefore, an outcome of evaluation more often than not is the decision that change needs to occur somewhere and to some degree in the curriculum. Stuffelbeam suggests that the decision to change occurs after contextual evaluation, when the faculty determines that change should be incremental (small), metamorphic (large) or neomobilistic (quick).

Stages of Change

If the faculty decides to change the curriculum based on its evaluation, there are three major stages of change according to Kelman's theory of social influence, Simpson's theory of socialization, and Schein's model of planned change that will become evident during the change process (Woolley, 1978).

STAGE I: COMPLIANCE TO CHANGE

Compliance to change involves an unfreezing process and an anticipating role expectation in the beginning phase of changing. During Stage I, the goal of the change-agents is to create within the population (faculty) the motivation to change. According to Lewin's force field analysis, the change-agents (1) create within the faculty a lack of confirmation of their present values, beliefs, and behavior patterns within the old curriculum, by (2) inducing anxiety in the faculty as the actual curriculum is compared with an ideal or proposed curriculum, and by (3) creating a psychologically safe environment for the change by decreasing threats posed by the advent of the planned new curriculum (Reading book, . . . in Human Relations Training, 1968).

Compliance is the outcome of the unfreezing. The result of compliance is that faculty allows itself to be influenced.

TABLE 12. SUMMARY OF EVALUATION MODELS

	Decision Making (Stuffelbeam)	Countenance (Stake)	Behavioral Objectives (Tyler)	Goal-free (Scriven)
Purpose	To provide information for decision making	To describe and judge programs	To determine extent objectives have been reached	To judge multiple effects and merits of program
Key emphasis	Decision making	Judgments based on descriptive data	Measurement of attainment of outcomes	Combining data of different weights (effects)
Method	Surveys, questionnaires, interviews	Case studies, interviews, observations	Achievement tests, tests, and measurements	Logical analysis of data, conceptual analysis
Outcomes	Quality control	Understanding	Accountability	Social utility
Major audience	Administrators, decision makers	Teachers, administrators	Teachers, managers	Consumers
Typical questions	Is the program effective?	What does the program look like to different people?	Are the objectives being achieved? Is the teacher producing?	What are all the effects?

Design implication	Nonexperimental Four areas (CIPP) always including delineation of data, obtaining and reporting data	Very general matrices	Empiric design based on behavioral objectives	Formative and summative factors
Evaluation	Relevant, objective pervasive	Panoramic, descriptive, and judgmental	Related to behavioral objectives	Wholistic
Strengths	Supplies data for decision makers Allows evaluation to take place at any stage in program Wholistic	Systematic method for arranging descriptive and judgmental data	Easy	Discriminates between formative and summative Delineation of different types and weights of evaluation
Limitations	Maybe costly and complex Decision-making process unclear Method of data delineation ill-defined	Not clear what data are to be collected and how Some cells of data matrix overlap	Tendency to oversimplify evaluation process Focus on terminal objectives or summative evaluation Focus of attainment of objectives not on worth of objectives	What data should be Primary? Secondary? Tertiary? Limited methodology in the judging process

(Adapted from Worthen and Sanders, 1973; House, 1978.)

STAGE II: IDENTIFICATION WITH THE CHANGE
Identification with the change is the second stage. As change occurs there becomes an attachment by the more reticent faculty to significant others (peers) involved in the new curriculum. The "converted" faculty starts to add to its own behavior, behaviors reflecting an interest and belief in the proposed change. The goal or outcome of identification with the change is the development of new beliefs within the faculty.

STAGE III: INTERNALIZATION OF THE CHANGE
Refreezing is the internalization of the change by faculty. Faculty believes in the new curriculum or proposed changes and integrates them into its own value system. The goal or outcome is a stabilization and integration within faculty and the program of the new beliefs.

Behaviors of Change

During the three stages of change, an array of behaviors can and will be exhibited by faculty. Bogart (1977) lists such behaviors in an adaptation framework based on a passive–aggressive continuum.

1. Withdrawal: Some faculty will passively approach the proposed change by way of escape.
2. Denial: Some faculty will remain in the threatening environment, but will develop a block in receiving threatening input (proposed changes) from that environment.
3. Splitting: Some faculty will negatively adapt to the proposed change by forming different committees or informal subgroups which have the potential of diffusing the mission of the proposed change.
4. Substitution: Instead of pursuing the plan of the proposed change, there may be faculty that wants to propose a substitution plan or a plan to determine whether the proposed plan has credibility.
5. Problem solving: Some faculty will choose problem solving as a method of adaptation. In the problem-solving approach, there is a realistic assessment of the proposed change, which includes assessment of resources, realistic and worthwhile goals, priority setting, action-strategy planning, and execution of plan and evaluation.
6. Aggression: The last behavior on the passive–aggressive continuum is aggression. Faculty's (or administration's) method in aggression is to employ attack strategies in order to force the proposed change upon the faculty.

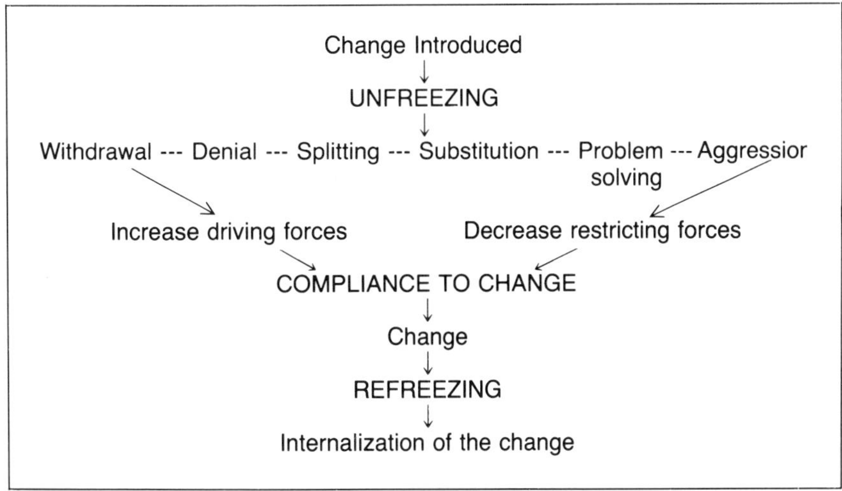

Figure 40. Process of change.

Planned Change

Since change is a dynamic balance or imbalance of all these passive–aggressive forces within the social-psychological space of the institution, planned change has to occur. Recognizing that the three major change stages will be occurring, faculty might take into consideration Lewin's three major strategies for achieving change: increasing the driving forces, decreasing the restraining forces, or both (Reading book, . . . in Human Relations Training, 1968). If increasing the driving forces is the only planned change strategy employed by faculty, tension in the system will be increased. Decreasing the restraining forces reduces opposition and thereby possibly increases the driving forces by default. Planned change requires work, intensive work, by the change-agents. One-to-one conferences and small group meetings for the purpose of discussion are strategies for reducing resisting forces and unfreezing, as well as defusing tensions. As the driving forces are increased, committees form to conduct the proposal and change will begin. Eventually, change will be accomplished and refreezing will be simultaneous with the new curriculum implementation (Fig. 40).

Evaluation is continuous and forever. Change is never ending. Evaluation procedures can be a headache, confusing, and disorganized. Evaluation can be organized and systematic through the use of existing models and thus lead to a fairly systematic organized outcome of stabilization or revision of the curriculum.

REFERENCES

Bogart, D. W. *Adaptive mechanism hierarchies in social systems*. Paper presented at Indiana University School of Nursing, 1977.

Clark, T., Goodwin, M., Mariani, et al. Curriculum evaluation: An application of Stuffelbeam's model in a baccalaureate school of nursing. *J Nurs Educ,* 1983, 22, 54–58.

Clayton, E. R., & Triplett, J. I. Measuring effects of a liberal education. *Nurs Outlook,* 1981, 29, 582–585.

Ediger, J., Snyder, M., & Corcoran, S. Selecting a model for use in curriculum evaluation. *Nurs Educ,* 1983, 22, 224–227.

Fields, C. Nursing schools get low marks for efforts to recruit blacks. *Chron Higher Educ,* May 14, 1979, p. 15.

Flaskerud, J. Utilizing a nursing conceptual model in basic level curriculum development. *J Nurs Educ,* 1983, 22, 224–227.

Ford, C. & Morgan, M. K. (Eds.). *Teaching in the Health Professions*. St. Louis: C. V. Mosby, 1976.

House, E. R. Assumptions underlying evaluation models. *Educ Research,* 1978, 7, 4–12.

Marriner, A., Langford, T., & Goodwin, L. D. Curriculum evaluation: Wordfact, ritual or reality. *Nurs Outlook,* 1980, 28, 228–232.

Mays, R. Affirmative Action Representative. Personal communication. 1979.

McMorrow, M. E. Nursing faculty response to open-door policy. *J Nurs Educ,* 1978, 17, 32–34.

Melcolm, N., Venn, R., & Bausell, R. B. The prediction of state board test pool examination scores within the integrated curriculum. *J Nurs Educ,* 1981, 20, 24–28.

National League for Nursing. *Criteria for the Evaluation of Baccalaureate and Higher Degree Programs in Nursing* (5th ed.). New York: National League for Nursing Publication 15–1251, 1983.

National League for Nursing. *Criteria for the Evaluation of Educational Programs in Nursing Leading to an Associate Degree* (5th ed.). New York: National League for Nursing Publication 23–1258, 1982.

National League for Nursing. *Program evaluation*. New York: National League for Nursing Publication 15–1738, 1978.

Packard, K. L., Schwebel, A. I., & Ganey, J. S. Concerns of final semester baccalaureate nursing students. *Nurs Research,* 1979, 28, 302–304.

Reading book. *Twenty-second Annual Laboratories in Human Relations Training 1968–1969*. Washington, D. C.: NTL Institute for Applied Behavioral Science Associated with the National Education Association, 1968.

Steele, S. *Educational Evaluation in Nursing*. USA: Charles B. Slack, 1978.

Stroller, E. P. Preconceptions of the nursing role: A case study of an entering class. *J Nurs Educ,* 1978, 17, 2–13.

Woolley, A. S. From RN to BSN: Faculty perceptions. *Nurs Outlook*, 1978, 26, 103–107.

Worthen, B. R., & Sanders, J. R. *Educational Evaluation: Theory and Practice*. Worthington, Ohio: Charles A. Jones, 1973.

Yess, J. P. Predictions of success in community college nursing education. *J Nurs Educ*, 1980, 19, 19–24.

9

Conclusion of Unit 3

AN EXAMPLE OF PRODUCT EVALUATION FOR RECYCLING DECISIONS

Questions Asked for Data Gathering	*Sources of Data*
What evaluation model should faculty use?	1. Literature review 2. Worthen and Sanders (1973)
Are the students meeting the objectives of the program?	1. Number of graduates compared to number of admissions 2. State board results 3. Success of graduates employed/in graduate school 4. Survey of seniors as to whether they think they have met objectives 5. Survey of graduates to determine if they feel now they had met the objectives upon graduation 6. Survey of graduates' supervisors
Did integration occur in the graduates?	1. Small group discussion between faculty and students with questions based on determining integration
Was the conceptual framework operationalized?	1. Peterson (1977)

How does the graduate compare to the predictors for program success?	1. Comparison of statistics on graduates' grades, employment, state board scores to predictors: SAT-V, SAT-M, EPPS, high school rank, GPA
What were the effects of liberal studies?	1. Clayton and Triplett's measurement tool (1981)
What was the success of minorities?	1. Statistics of numbers entering versus numbers graduating
What is the effectiveness of the program's administration?	1. Evaluation every 3 to 5 years 2. Evaluation by faculty, students, central administration 3. Evaluation tool for administrators (Ford and Morgan, 1976)
What is the effectiveness of teachers?	1. Evaluation every semester or year 2. Evaluation tool for teachers (Ford and Morgan, 1976) 3. Evaluation by students, peers, and administration
What is the effectiveness of the program?	1. Outreach meetings with clinical facility personnel 2. Faculty small group discussions comparing philosophy, objectives, and design with student progression, consumer needs, and professional organizations' position papers and resolutions
Is change necessary?	1. Data from measurement tools compared to existent program
What kind of change is necessary?	1. Context evaluation

RECYCLING DECISIONS

So, now we end (or do we begin?) with product evaluation. Data from product evaluation fuel context evaluation for a recycle of the whole program evaluation process. And you thought you were through.

Unit 4

GOVERNANCE

Without governance by someone or some group, chaos would be the name of the game for curricular planning. Governance provides an organization and structure for developing, structuring, implementing, and evaluating the curriculum.

10

Governance

There are three common elements in the nursing program's organization and governance. One element is the dean's office; a second is the faculty which usually does its business through a series of standing committees; and a third element is the structure by which the faculty organizes to do its daily work, a set of departments or units within the organization formed around activities or entities such as curricular levels, conceptual threads or subject matter (Redman and Barley, 1978).

COLLEGIAL ORGANIZATION AND GOVERNANCE

In a collegial democracy, the traditional organizational framework of the university, the powers of the dean and the faculty are in frequent interplay, a series of checks and balances (Redman et al., 1978; Styles, 1983). The authority–responsibility relationship within the domains of both faculty and administration is in general widely agreed upon. Deans have traditionally been held accountable by higher administration for the fiscal management of an academic unit as well as for supervising the set of operations by which the organization achieves its goals. Faculty has been held accountable for both policy recommendation and decision making in the areas of curriculum and instruction, educational policy, and research. In actuality there are many areas of overlap between the administrative and faculty domains, requiring a highly consultative style on the part of the administration and faculty sensitivity to institutional constraints, including the financial implications of curricular proposals and organizational demands. A collegial organization emphasizes the collaboration of the faculty with administration in the management of its own affairs, the faculty being aware of a differentiation of function and seeking consensus in a fully participatory manner (Styles, 1983).

Constitution and Bylaws

Since a collegiate organization is a dynamic entity and today exists in a situation of rapid change, a clear organizational conception needs to be articulated in a codified form. Such a document, the school's constitution and bylaws, establishes the processes in the collegial structure by which policies are created, put into practice, and reviewed. Since the aim of the document is to provide a guide for the day-to-day operation of the school, making the checks and balances actually function well, it is necessary for it to be clear and understandable (Redman et al., 1978).

The easiest way to avoid an ambiguous or incomplete constitution and bylaw document is to think in terms of the mission of the school or program when composing and interpreting it, rather than of tasks to be accomplished (Redman et al., 1978). The constitution defines the name and purpose of the organization, the membership, voting privileges, and other elements of the structure meant to be relatively permanent. Bylaws provide further details, such as committee structure, function, and membership. They include a parliamentary mechanism for their own alteration in order to adapt to developing situations without having to overhaul the whole constitution.

> Several issues are commonly of concern when constructing a document for governance of a school. One is the degree of delegation of power from the general faculty of standing committees; a second is breadth of scope of most committees; a third is the matter of representation. These are interrelated and are dependent on the competence of members, and on the school's sense of itself as a total body (Redman et al., 1978, p. 30).

GOVERNANCE

"What do faculty govern? . . . Faculty exercise control over matters relating to curriculum and instruction, research, faculty status, and educational policy" (Styles, 1983, p. 284).

By what right does faculty govern? By tradition, vested authority (such as state statutes, university bylaws, and policy manuals), expert authority in academic matters, and the application of that authority in appropriate behavior. More recently the process of negotiation has emerged as a new means of access to governance rights in the "dynamic, diverse, politically charged environment in which faculty roles are subject to the vicissitudes of changing priorities and pressures" (Styles, 1982, p. 285).

Influencing Variables on Governance

In such a dynamic situation, several variables can dramatically alter and influence the governance of a program. The same constitution and bylaws may function quite differently in two separate programs, for example, as the leadership style of the director, the philosophy of the program, or the nature of the institution differs (Styles, 1983; Marriner, 1980; Redman et al., 1978).

MODELS AND STYLES OF GOVERNANCE

Styles (1983) has identified three models of academic governance: the collegial, the bureaucratic, and the political. She suggests that aspects of all three are found in every academic institution. Each model throws light on how this complex institution actually functions in its governance process.

The *collegial* model is the original image of the college as a community of expert scholars managing its affairs in a round table manner without external interference, through the development of consensus.

The *bureaucratic* model describes the rational, efficient, goal-directed, organizational form of a school requiring explicit policies, decisions, and managerial direction.

The *political* model, more prominent in recent times, assumes conflict rather than consensus to be the normal state of affairs in any academic organization and takes into account phenomena such as interests, elites, divergent goals, and the struggle to control the decision-making process.

Each of these models generates a predominant style of governance, all having the possibility of being present in one program, depending on the tasks at hand (Marriner, 1980). Both the collegial and political styles are very participatory in nature while the bureaucratic style is more task-oriented and autocratic. Generally one style tends to predominate regardless of task, but the other two may periodically emerge as dominant depending on several variables within the system. When divergent goals and displeasure over the governance processes arise, various pressures will be brought to bear and the political aspects of relationships in the institution will predominate.

CONFLICT OF GOVERNANCE STYLES

Within an institution, whatever the organization and predominant type of governance, styles of governance are an important variable. The faculty may struggle to implement a collegial model of governance, but an autocratic dean or director will render this struggle futile unless the faculty changes the dean's methods or perhaps, deans. Even so, if the dean and faculty agreed to a collegial mode of governance but the rest of the institution were autocratic in its organization and ethos, there would not be a "goodness-of-fit," resulting in frustration on the part of the faculty and administration and a further dissipation of resources, especially time and energy, in the ensuing politicization.

A healthy governance system in a reasonably mature collegiate situation will provide an environment conducive to collegiality with functioning mechanisms in which real or potential conflicts can be aired and mediated (Styles, 1983; Marriner, 1980). Strong administration and managerial leadership will keep it that way.

GOVERNANCE AND CURRICULUM

Whatever its structure, the organization and governance of the program is the setting in which the curriculum is developed, implemented, and evaluated. Yet as a result of that structure the curriculum is owned or disowned, honored or dishonored, respected or disrespected by the faculty.

The curriculum belongs to the faculty; it is the expression of the will and the mind of the faculty. It is the main vehicle for carrying out the philosophy and vocation of the teacher.

When faculty has not shaped and reshaped the curriculum and cannot look forward to its continuing review in the light of its experience with it and the development of new knowledge, there will seldom be a sense of ownership and respect for it, and consequently its implementation is in jeopardy. Faculty that has developed the curriculum because of and within the organization and governance of its program will own, honor, and respect the curriculum and will aggressively and actively implement it.

REFERENCES

Marriner, A. *Guide to Nursing Management*. St. Louis: C. V. Mosby, 1980.

Redman, B. K., & Barley, Z. A. On the governance system of university schools of nursing. *J Nurs Educ*, 1978, 17, 27–31.

Styles, M. M. Faculty governance. In M. E. Conway & O. Andruskin (Eds.), *Administrative Theory and Practice*. Norwalk, Connecticut: Appleton-Century-Crofts, 1983.

Index